Livestock Production Management
– A Practical Manual
(As per VCI Syllabus 2016, Paper 1)

Dr. Asma Khan
Associate Professor, Division of LPM

Dr. B. Brahma
Asst. Professor, Division of LPM

Dr. Dipanjali Konwar
Asst. Professor, Division of LPM

Dr. Manpreet Kour
Asst. Professor, Division of ILFC

SKUAST - JAMMU, R.S. PURA-181 102, J&K

SSPH

SATISH SERIAL PUBLISHING HOUSE
403, Express Tower, Commercial Complex
Azadpur, Delhi-110033 (India)
Phone : 011-27672852, Fax : 91-11-27672046
e-mail : info@satishserial.com, hkjain1975@yahoo.com
Website : www.satishserial.com

Published by :

SATISH SERIAL PUBLISHING HOUSE
403, Express Tower, Commercial Complex, Azadpur, Delhi-110033 (INDIA)
Phone : 011-27672852 Fax : 91-11-27672046
E-mail : info@satishserial.com, hkjain1975@yahoo.com

ISBN 978-93-86200-53-2

Composed, Designed & Printed in India

Livestock Production Management
– A Practical Manual
(As per VCI Syllabus 2016, Paper 1)

Foreword

Livestock production systems worldwide need to be able to combine profitability with the responsibility of protecting human health, animal health, animal welfare and the environment. The Guide contains many individual practices that contribute to good dairy farming practice, covering the key aspects of animal health, milk hygiene, nutrition, welfare, the environment and socio-economic management. Compiling this information in form of a practical manual has vital academic importance. It gives me immense pleasure to know that Division of Livestock Production & Management has published a practical manual on recent scientific guidelines of livestock production management. The information provided in this manual shall serve as a ready reference and will make easy the students to follow and perform the practical in orderly manner especially unit IInd"Fodder production and conservation" which is a good attempt of its kind for the use of undergraduate students of B.V.Sc & AH.

I am confident that this manual, prepared as per new Veterinary council of India's recent guidelines and syllabus 2016, will be of immense help to the students of B. V. Sc. & A. H.

I value and worth the efforts made by the authors in preparation of this manual.

Prof. MMS Zama
Dean
F. V. Sc. & A. H.
SKUAST-Jammu

Preface

The ideas presented in this manual were gleaned from various sources and the authors' practical experience. The content of this manual has been planned keeping in consideration of new syllabus of B. V. Sc. & A. H. recommended by Veterinary Council of India (2016).

Livestock Production Management is an enormous subject and management practices could vary from place to place within the country. However, basic principles of livestock production management remain unchanged and should adhere to the conclusive results of various research outcomes. The content in this manual are based on research materials as well as standard methods described by eminent scientists.

The manual is written in simple language and style to give information which is essential and practical. The chapters in the manual are arranged in most logical manner. The selected questions at the end of the each chapter will be of help to the students. We shall welcome suggestions and healthy criticism of teachers and students for improving this manual.

Deeply felt gratitude is due to the Dean, F.V.Sc and A.H. SKUAST-J for inspiration and guidance as well as the financial support. Sincere thanks are also due to colleagues and friends for their constant help and encouragement.

We sincerely hope that this document will contribute in easy learning of the students.

Authors

Contents

1

Visit to the Livestock Farms and Identification of Breeds (Cattle, Buffalo, Sheep and Goats)

Date:

Objective

1. To get familiarize with the farm routine and the physical facilities available.
2. To get familiarize with the different species of livestock (Cattle Buffalo, Sheep and Goat) and their breeds available at the farm.

Material required

Live animals of different species, Models, charts, diagrams of different species, different physical facilities and Records/information on different aspects.

Procedure:

After taking a round of the livestock farms tabulate the following information:

1. Total allocated for fodder production.
2. Area allocated for fodder production.
3. Area under buildings.
4. Livestock species observed.
5. Name the breeds of each species and their objectives
6. Major schemes for different species and their objectives.
7. Type of housing systems.
8. Type of house for different categories of livestock.
9. Type of fodder available in different seasons.

10. Fodder conservation techniques.
11. Total milk and other products produced and their disposal.
12. Category wise livestock strength.
13. Feeding schedule for different categories.
14. Methods of milking.
15. Health care- vaccination schedule.

Precautions

1. Dip your feet in footbath if provided.
2. Don't try to tease or provoke the animals.
3. Don't make noise in the milking parlor.

Questions

1. Name the best breed of cattle and buffalo in India and World.
2. Which breed of exotic cattle gives the maximum milk per lactation?
3. Name the cattle breed whose milk is rich in milk fat.
4. What is the amount of maximum milk produced in a day by an animal in India as well as in the world?
5. Differentiate wet average from overall average with the help of an example.
6. Name a few crossbreds developed in India.

Signature of Teacher

❑❑❑

2

External Body Points of Different Livestock Species

Date:

Objective

1. To get familarise with the phenotypic body points of livestock species.
2. To describe and write the history sheet of the animal.
3. To explain the animals in the show rings.

Material required

Live animals, Models, charts, diagrams and Restraining equipment including crush, ropes, measuring tape, pointer etc.

Procedure

Before discussing body points on an animals, student must know

Left side	Vs	Right side
Dorsal	Vs	Ventral side
Front	Vs	Rear side

Then, body points can be discussed under five major headings veterinary students should be able to describe all these points.

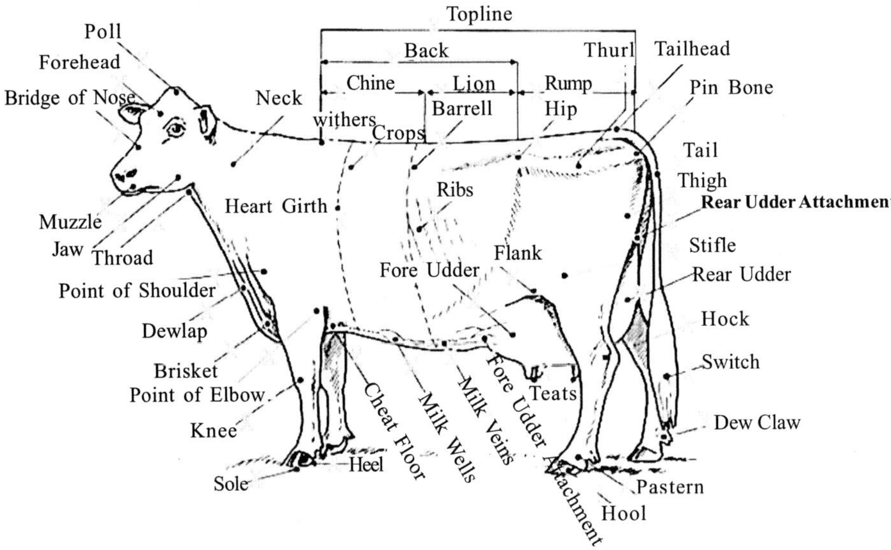

Parts of the Dairy Cow

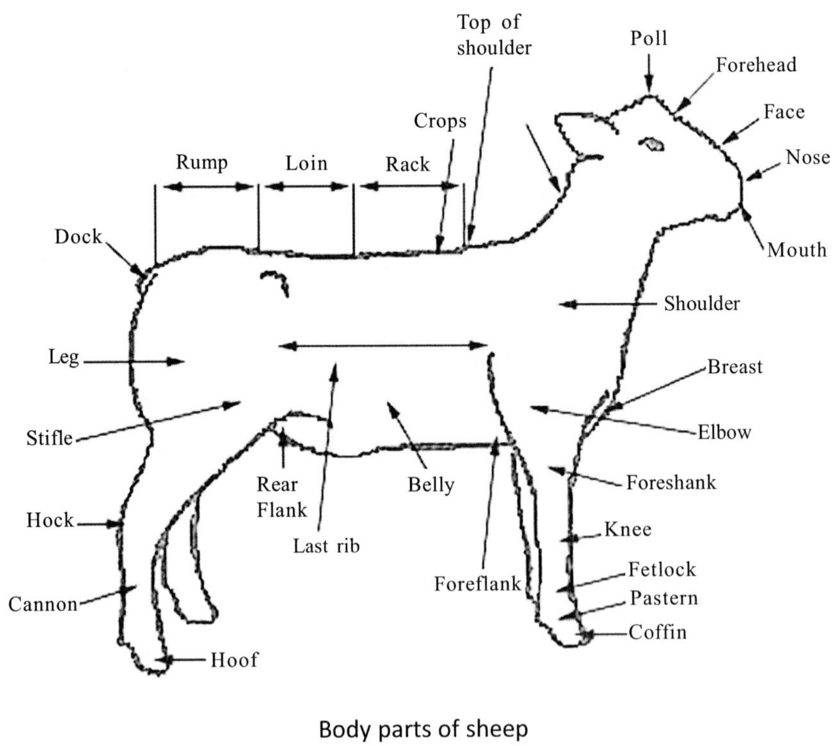

Body parts of sheep

Graphic Source : Web Resource

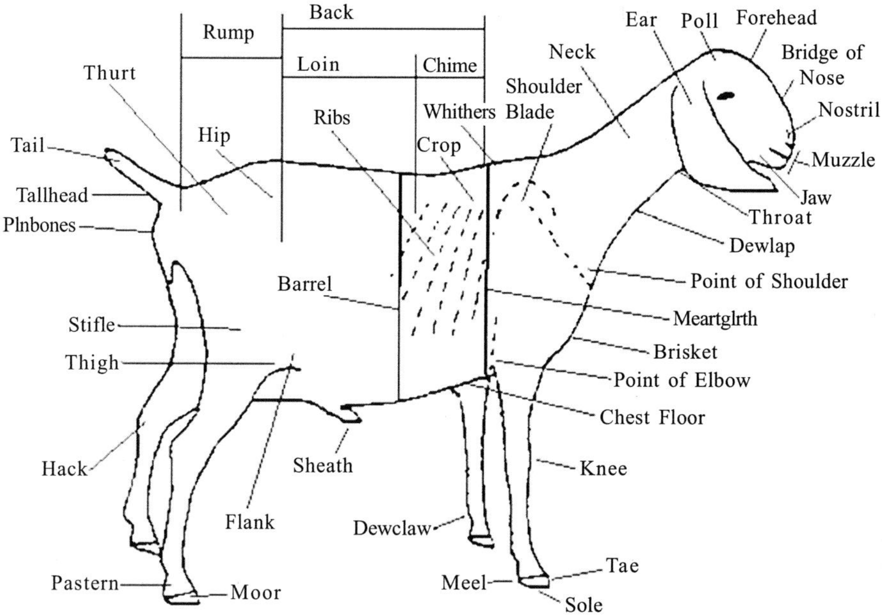

Body parts of goat

Graphic Source : Web Resource

Part of the head: These points are to be explained in anti-clockwise direction poll, horns, ears, eyes, temporal fossa, for head, face bridge of nose, cheeks, nostrils, jaws, muffle, mouth, chin, muzzle, jowl, throat.

Part of the neck: These points are to be explained in clockwise direction Apex of neck, crest, base of neck, hollow of the neck, dewlap, body of neck, jugular groove.

Parts of the trunk: These points are to be explained in clock wise direction starting from hump, withers, back, chine, loin, hip, rump pin bone, base of tail, body of tail, switch, anus, vulva (in females only), escutcheon point, udder, teats, milk vein, milk well, naval flap, prepuce, scrotum (in males), belly, abdominal region, flank, folds, chest, thoracic region, ribs, brisket, barrel, croup, thurl.

Parts of Forelimb: These points are to be explained from top to region bottom shoulder blade, point of shoulder, elbow, axilla, forearm, knee joint, shin/shank/cannon, fetlock joint, pastern, claws, toe, heel and sole.

Parts of Rearlimb: These points are to be explained from top to bottom where most of the points are same as of foreleg except thigh, buttocks, twist, groin, stifle and hock joint.

Precautions

1. Do not tease or hurt the animals while working on them.
2. Avoid carrying of a stick while working on animals.
3. Always describe the body points in a systematic manner.

Assignments

1. Prepare a comparative table of body points of cattle, buffalo, sheep, and goat.
2. Prepare a comparative table correlating the phenotypic body points with anatomical features of the skeleton.
3. Draw the sketch/line diagram of cow and label only those points.
4. Draw the sketch of buffalo, sheep and goat and label only those points which are different than of cow.

Questions

1. Why is it important to know the body points of an animal?
2. What is there in the milk vein?
3. What is the importance of milk well?
4. Indicate the most important difference between Indian and European cattle.

Signature of Teacher

□□□

3

Identification of Common Tools used on Animal Farm

Date:

Objective

1. To get familiarize with the common tools used in dairy farm operation.
2. To know the use of these tools in various farm operation.
3. To acquainted with the procedure of using the tools.

Material required

Live animals, Models, and different tools used in animal farm.

Procedure

Use of common tools used on animal farm are given below:

AI gun:Artificial Insemination

Balling gun: Medication (Bolus)

Body brush: Grooming of Animals

Dandy brush: Grooming of Animals

Hot branding rod: Identification

Freeze branding rod: Identification

Tattooing forceps: Identification

Ear tag piercer: Identification

Hoof trimmer: trimming of hooves

Bull nose puncture: fitting bull ring

Bull nose ring: Restraining

Bull holder: restraining

Electric debudder: disbudding

Burdizzo castrator: castration

Tail docker: docking

Drenching pipe: medication (liquid)

Drenching bottle: medication (liquid)

Probang gag: opening or oral cavity

Butler's gag:opening or oral cavity

Drinkwater gag: opening or oral cavity

Teat dip: disinfection of teats

Strip cup: Test for mastitis

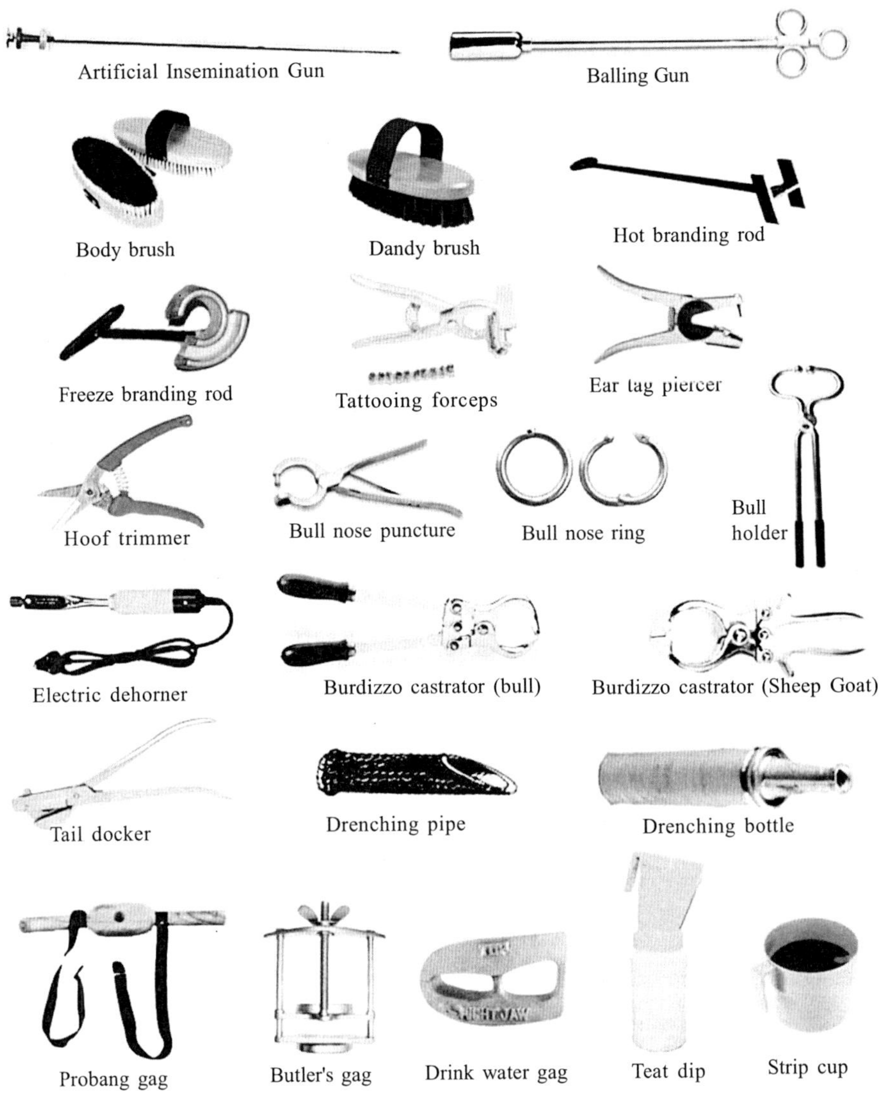

Graphic Source : Web Resource

Question

1. Identify the tools in the laboratory and write its use.

Signature of Teacher

❑❑❑

4

Familiarization with different knots used in controlling of animals

Date:

Objective

To approach, handle and restrain an animal for different managemental practices to be carried on the animal.

Principles of approaching and handling

Material Required

Animals, bull nose ring, bull nose punch, bull holder, bull leader, muzzle, ropes of different sizes and crush.

Prerequisite

Basic knowledge regarding general behaviour of the species/ animal to be handled.

Procedure

While restraining animals, it is important to be familiar with the handling of rope. The parts of the rope are, end and standing part. The end is a short piece and the standing part a large piece. A "bight" is formed after doubling a rope and a "loop" after a complete circle. While restraining the animal, a rope is secured by knots and hitches. A knot is an inter-twinning or tying together the pieces of rope or ropes. A hitch is temporary fastening of a rope to a post, hook or a fixed object. Various types of knots and hitches in common use are as follows:

a) **Overhand knot:** The end of one rope is crossed over and around the ends of the same rope over and around each other. The two ends are pulled to make a knot.

b) **Square knot:** Square knot is the ideal knot and is applied by first tying an overhand knot and then by crossing the right and over and around the left to make a second overhand knot, which is then tied.

c) **Surgeon's Knot:** The end of the one rope is crossed over and around the end of the other rope and one more turn of the end is taken around the standing the part. Further, the end is crossed on the right over and around the left end and is pulled tight.

d) **Slip knot:** A loop is made in the end of the rope and is placed over the standing part the end is passes behind the standing part and upward through the loop. The end is pulled tight to make a slip knot.

e) **Granny's knot:** The end of the left rope is crossed over and around the end of the right rope, as in square knot. Later the new left rope is crossed over and then around new right rope. The knot is secured tightly. Granny's knot is not preferred since it will slip under strain whereas square knot will hold firmly.

f) **Bowline:** A loop is made in the standing part of the rope, then the end is passed through the loop and over the standing part. The end is caught after reaching under the standing part and is brought under it and then through the loop. The end and both the standing parts are pulled to tie the knot.

Commonly used hitches are:

Half Hitch

i) **Single half hitch:** The end of the rope is taken around the object and is brought over and then under the standing part. It is pulled to form a single half hitch.

ii) **Double half hitch:** A single half hitch is applied and then second single half hitch over the standing part of the rope. The standing part and the end are pulled to tie the knot.

Clove hitch

The center part of the rope is grasped with both hands and the hands are rotated an counter-clockwise direction to form two loops. The loops are brought together so that the right loop overlaps the left one. The ends of the rope are pulled to make the clove hitch.

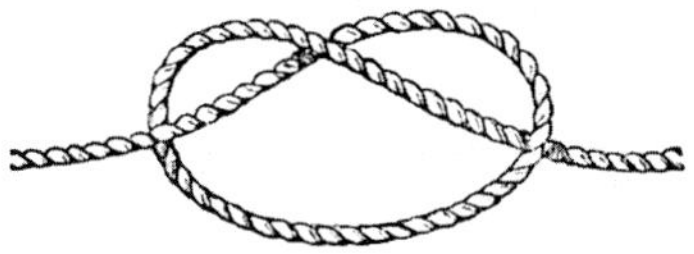

Overhand knot

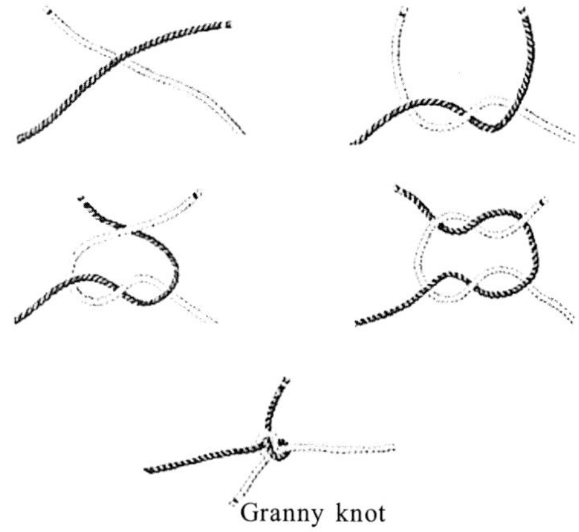

Granny knot

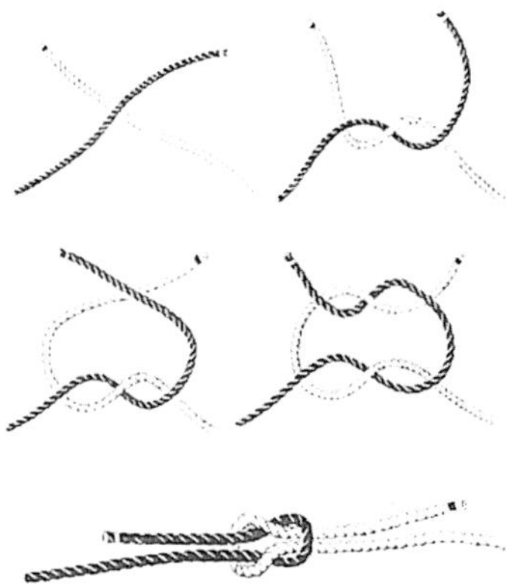

Square knot

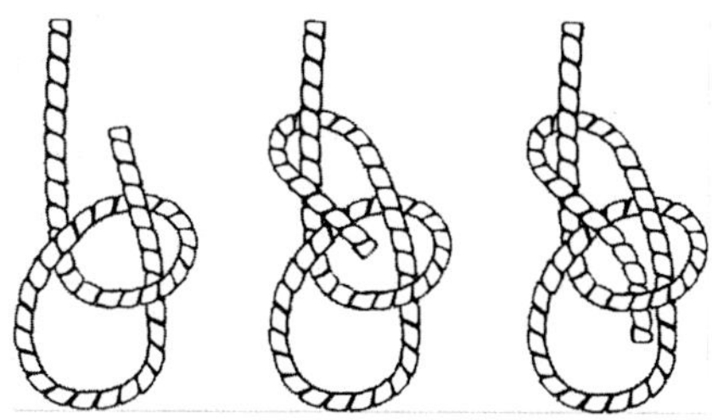

Bowline knot

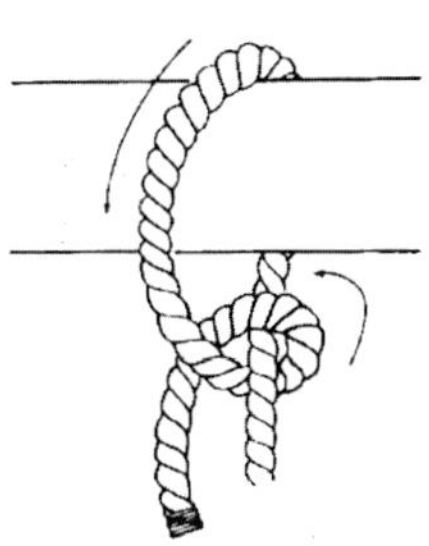

Half hitch

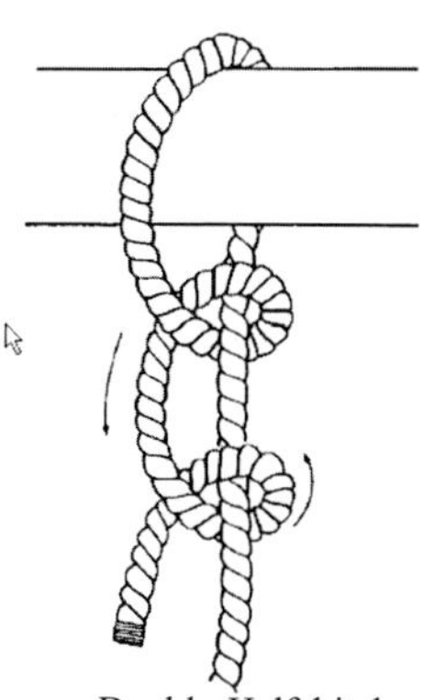

Double Half hitch

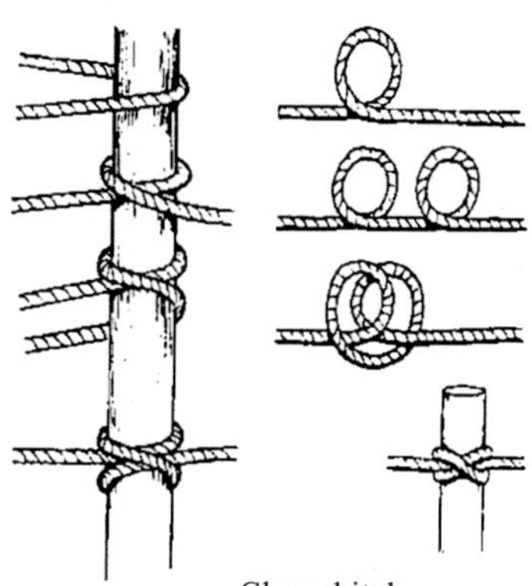

Clove hitch

Graphics Compiled and edited from Web Resources

Assignments

a) Practice and write the procedure for application of all knots in general and milkman's knot, halter, straight jacket and casting ropes in particular. Also mention the length and thickness of ropes required.

b) Draw the diagrams of various equipments required for the above said exercise.

Questions

a) What are the functions of different knots, hitches and splices?

Signature of Teacher

❑❑❑

5

Methods of Identification in Animals

Date:

Objective

a) To establish the ownership

b) To maintain various records like history sheet, growth, reproduction, production and health cards etc.

Material required

Depends on the method followed/required.

Tagging: Ear tag, tag applicator, neck tags along with chain.

Tattooing: Tattooing machine, tattooing number, tattooing ink, scissor, spirit, cotton.

Branding: Branding number, angithi.

Notching: Notching forceps.

In addition to the above said techniques for the identification there are many other methods e.g.:

- Leg and wing bands - commonly applied in poultry birds.
- Body numbers/paints
- Hair whorls
- Photographs/sketches
- Colour devices
- Electronic identification with RFID tags

Procedure

Ear tags: They may be of plastic or metal. Select a site on the left ear in such a way that it does not have any prominent vein. Fix the tag in the tag applicator or tagging machine so that when it is applied in the ear it can be easily read from left to right.

Neck tags: It may be of cardboard, plastic, aluminum which can be tied around the neck with the help of neck chain.

Tattooing: It is generally done in the young age. Clean the left ear from inner side with spirit. Remove the surplus hair. Fix the required number in the tattooing machine. Apply tattooing ink and tattoo the predetermined number keeping the following precautions in mind:

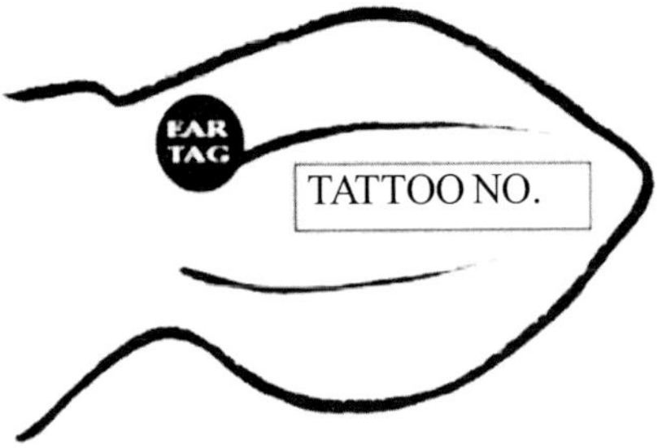

- Try to select the area which is light in colour.
- Prominent veins should not be punctured.
- Restrain the animal properly at the time of tattooing.
- Check the number on a piece of paper before its final application.

Branding: It can be of two types:

- Hot branding
- Cold branding

Generally branding is done at about 2 years of age in cattle and buffalo. In hot branding, after casting the animal on the ground, the red hot brand number is applied on the left thigh of the animal.

In cold branding, the brand number are dipped in the liquid nitrogen at -196° C and applied on the thigh similarly as in the case of hot branding. Both have the burning effect. Brand numbers are available both in alphabets and numerals.

Ear Notching: Ear notching is widely used in the swine industry as a system of animal identification. Ear notching involves removing V shaped portions of the ear that correspond to a specific litter number and also an individual pig number from that litter. There are many systems of ear notching, but usually the litter number is notched in the pig's right ear, and the individual pig number is notched in the pig's left ear. The notches are numbered from the bottom of the ear, with the number one being next to the head. Multiplying this number by three will give the next notch number (*i.e.*, 3, 9, 27) which is adjacent to the area where the previous notch was located. Start at the bottom of the ear next to the head and continue to the top of the ear, then work back toward the head. The exception to this is the tip of the right ear, which is the position for the 81-notch. Pigs must be notched within 7 days of birth.

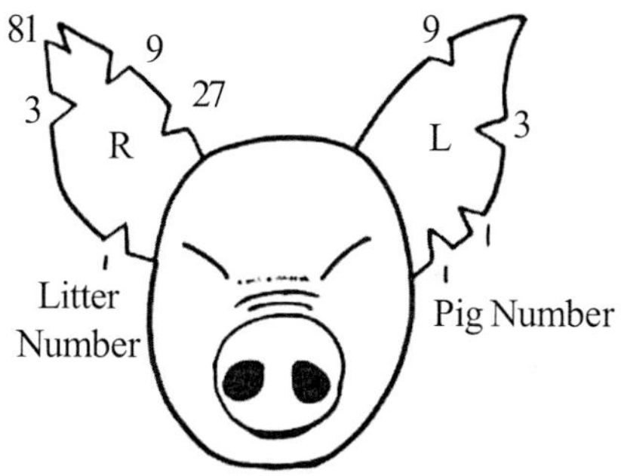

PIG No. 121-14

Precautions

All the methods are not applicable for all species therefore firstly decide the methods to be used on a particular species and according to its age group.

Animals can also be identified by keeping a record of their natural marks spots, patches body colours, chestnuts, acquired marks-scars of wounds etc., or photographs.

Comparative merits and demerits of different methods of marking:

S.No	Parameters	Tattooing	Branding	Tagging
1.	Marking permanent	Yes	Yes	No
2.	Number seen from distance	No	Yes	Yes
3.	Reduces quality of hide	No	Yes	No
4.	Suitable on dark animals	No	Yes	Yes
5.	Species commonly used	Cattle Sheep Goat	Buffaloes Cattle Cattle	Cattle Sheep Goat

Assignments

Draw the diagrams of different equipment used by different techniques for identification.

Questions

1. Why branding is not done in sheep and goat?

2. Which is the most appropriate method of identification in calves?
3. For permanent marking, which methods you will follow and why?
4. Name the different methods you will use to cast cattle and buffaloes?
5. Why spirit is used for cleaning ears?

Signature of Teacher

❑❑❑

6

Ageing, Weighing and Measurements of Farm Animals

Date:

Objective

- To know the growth and development of the animal.
- Comparison of animals in the show ring.
- Transaction of animals.
- To ascertain the age in Vet- legal cases.

Material required

Ready reckoners for ageing, weighing balance, measuring tape, animals and restraining equipment.

Procedure

AGEING: Age can be ascertained either by

i) Records – Actual date of birth

ii) General appearance

iii) Horn rings

iv) Dentition

Age determination by dentition

After birth records, dentition is the most reliable method of age estimation. In the beginning age can be estimated from eruption of deciduous teeth, then from permanent teeth and ultimately from wear and tear along with change in the shape, coloration, size of the teeth.

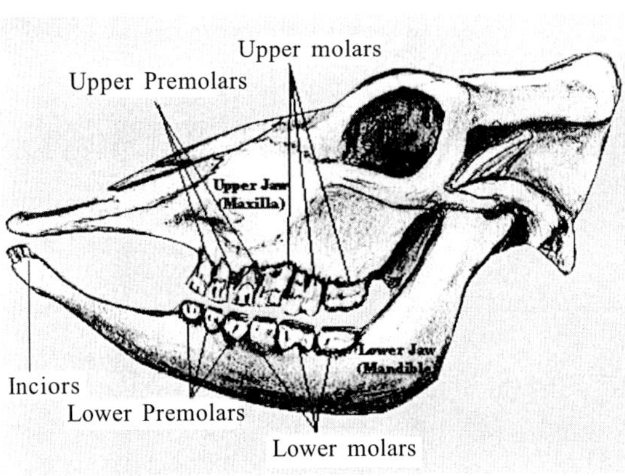

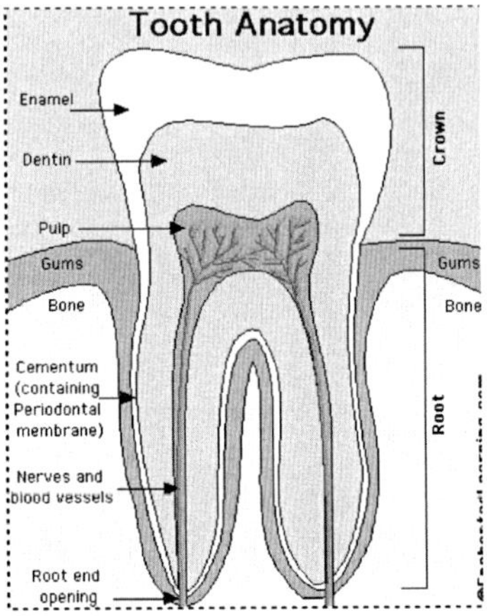

Graphic Source : Web Resource

Types of Teeth

Temporary teeth: These are present at birth or may erupt during after birth, but later pushed out by the growth of corresponding permanent teeth. Temporary teeth occurs only in incisors and premolars. Temporary teeth are small, white with a distinct neck.

Permanent teeth: These teeth appears at a certain age and remain in them throughout the life of animal. Permanent teeth are larger, stronger, browner in colour and has no marked neck.

Common terms related to dentition

Alveolus: The follow cavity of jaw bones in which the root of a tooth is embedded.

Canine teeth: One pair of sharp teeth situates next to corner incisors of each jaw of some species. These are also known as tusks. (in Pig) and touch (horses).

Crown: The part of teeth that appears above the gum.

Dental Pad: The hard pad of the upper jaw of bovine in place of the incisors.

Full Mouth: When all permanent teeth have fully erupted. However it is consider to only the incisors.

Cheek teeth: Premolars and molars together known as cheek teeth.

Surface: Outer surface cheek teeth.

Labial: The surface of the tooth nut to the lips.

Lingual: The surface of the tooth nut to the tongue.

Table or wearing surface: That surface of the tooth which grinds the food and comes in contact with similar surface of corresponding tooth of the other jaw.

In wear: Means that the whole of the table of a tooth is in contact with the opposing tooth or teeth of the other jaw.

In cattle and buffalo beyond 8 years and small animals (Sheep & Goat) beyond 5 years are generally termed as aged animal without trying estimated the exact age.

Broken Mouthed: Aged animal when one or more teeth fallen is called broken mouthed.

Gummers are Animals in which all teeth have fallen are called gummers

Mark: The mark is the blackened depression which is seen on the table. It is lined by a distinct, narrow, pearly white ring of enamel. In the new tooth the mark is very broad and deep, but with the age and wear, it becomes shallower and smaller, till it finally disappears altogether. Enamel is stands up a little above the level of the rest of the surface.

Neck: The point where the gum and tooth meet is the neck.

Fang: Is the part of the tooth within the jaw. It is hollow and its cavity (fang hole) contains the blood vessels and nerves which nourish and supply nerve to the tooth. As the tooth grows up, the fang hole becomes filled in with tooth substances of a lighter colour than the remainder and when the wear reaches this level, it appears on the lable of the tooth as a small white spot in the center, or in front of the mark. If that has not already disappear.

DENTAL FORMULAE

Species	Temporary	Permanent
Cattle, Buffalo	0030	0033
Sheep, Goat	4030	4033
Camel	1030	1133
	3020	3123
Swine	3040	3143
	3040	3143

Dentition chart of cattle, buffalo, sheep goat and pig:

Teeth	Cow	Sheep and Goat	Pig
Di 1	Before birth	0–1 wk	3–4 wk
Di 2	Before birth	1–2 wk	2–3 months
Di 3	0–1 wk	2–3 wk	Before birth
I 1	2 yr	1–1 ½ yr	12–15 months
I 2	2 ½ yr	1 ½–2 yr	16–20 months
I 3	3 ½ yr	2–2 ½ yr[b]	8–10 months
Dc/Di 4[a]	0–2 wk	3–4 wk	Before birth
I4/C	3 ½–4 yr	2 ½–4 yr[c]	6–10 months
Dp 2	0–3 wk	0–4 wk	4–6 wk
Dp 3	0–3 wk	0–4 wk	1 ½ months
Dp 4	0–3 wk	0–4 wk	1–5 wk
P 1	–	–	5 months
P 2	2–2 ½ yr	1 ½–2 yr	12–15 months
P 3	2–2 ½ yr	1 ½–2 yr	12–15 months
P 4	2 ½–3 yr	1 ½–2 yr	12–15 months
M 1	5–6 months	3–6 months[d]	4–6 months
M 2	1–1 ½ yr	9–12 months	8–12 months
M 3	2–2 ½ yr	1 ½–2 yr	18–20 months

[a] Di = deciduous incisor Dp = deciduous premolar Dc = deciduous canine [b] 2 yr in goats; [c] 2 ½–3 yr in goats; [d] 3–4 month in sheep

Determination of age through horn rings

As the horns grow in size with increase in age of animal, rings get formed on it. First ring on the horns appears at 3 years age in Zebu cattle, thereafter, every year a ring appears. Hence the following formula may be used.

$n + 2$ = Age of animal in years

n = number of rings on horns

Limitations

1. Removal of the rings in the horn with a rasp or oiling of the horn adds to the difficulty in determining correct age.

2. Rings are not clear on small horns in some breeds.
3. Present trend is to keep animals dehorned, hence this method cannot be used in dehorned or polled animals.

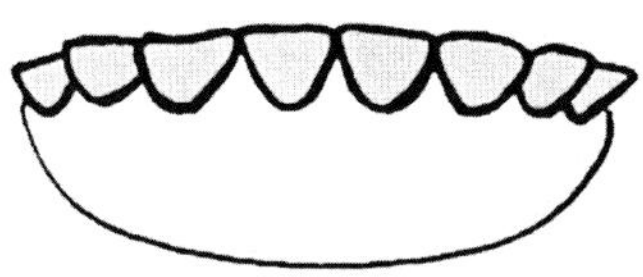

Milk tooth: about 0 to 24 months

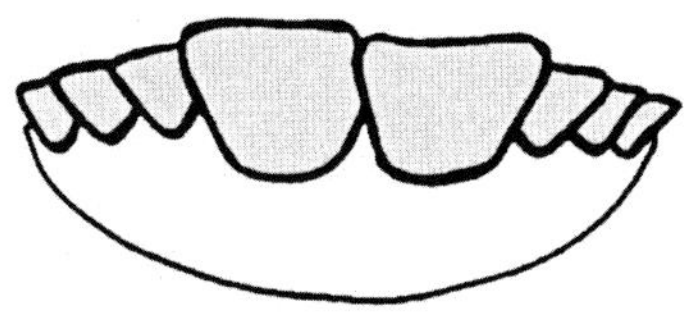

2-tooth: about 18 to 30 months

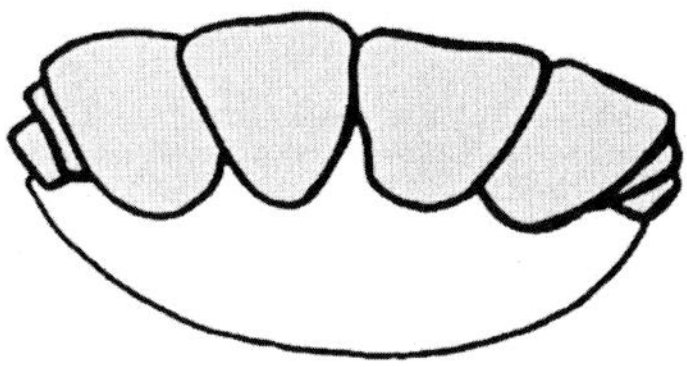

4-tooth: about 24 to 36 months

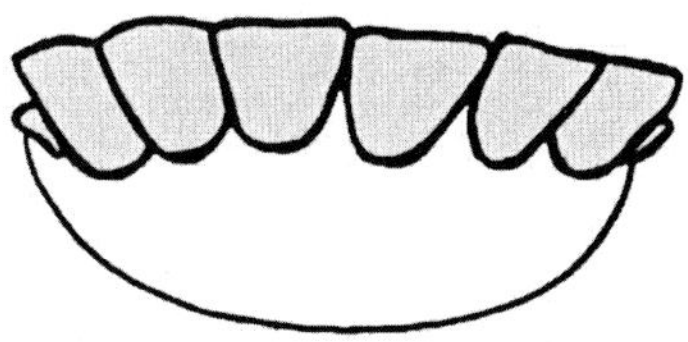

6-tooth: about 30 to 42 months

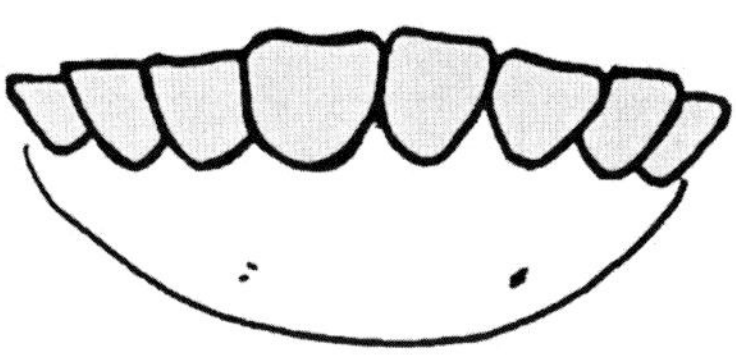

8-tooth: about 36 months onwards

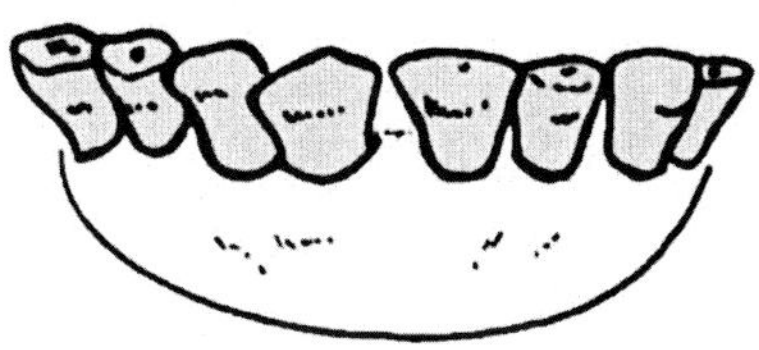

Worn full mouth: from about 7 years

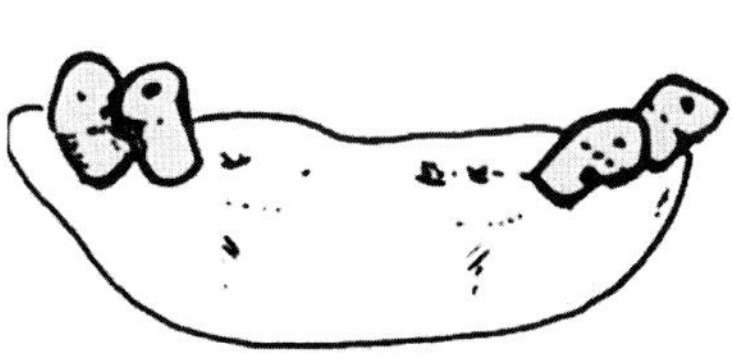

Broken mouth: from about 8 years

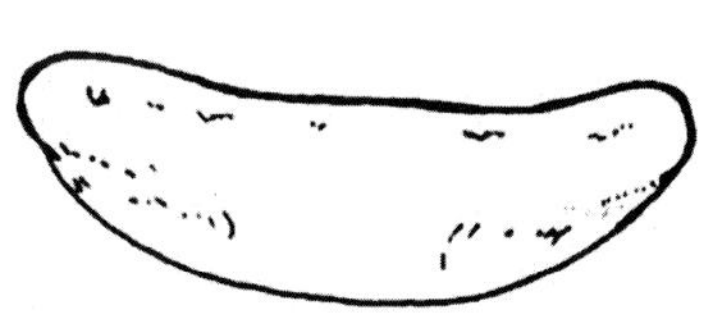

Gummv mouth: from about 9 years

Dentition chart of cattle

Graphic Compiled and edited from Web Resource

Estimation of weight

The weight of the animal is essential for the following purposes:

1. To find out the status of health of animal
2. To study the weight gain during experiments.
3. For computation of rations.
4. For calculating the correct dosage of medicine.

Direct method

Usually animals are weighted once in a month.

1. **Weighing bridge:** The animal is made to stand on the plateform of the weighing bridge and it records the weight in pounds (lb) or kilogram (Kg)
2. **Spring balance:** Sheep and goat may be weighed by using the spring balance.
3. **Platform balance:** Small ruminants can be weighed by using plateform balance.

Indirect method

1. By using formula

Shaffer's formula

This is the most common formula used for cattle and buffaloes. This formula tends to under-estimate weight of very young and very heavy animals.

$W = LG^2 / 300$

In this formula the weight of the animal is expressed in pounds.

Where,

L = Length of the animal from point of shoulder to point of buttocks in inches.

G = chest girth of the animal in inches.

Minnesota formula

$W = LG^2 / 600$

In this formula the weight of animal is expressed in kilograms.

Where,

L is the length of the animal from point of shoulder to point of buttocks in inches.

G is the chest girth of the animal in inches.

Agarwal's modified Shaffer's formula

Formula for Indian cattle is as follows

Live weight in seers = Girth x length / Y

Where Y is equal to 9.0 if girth is less than 65 inches

Y is equal to 8.5 if girth is between 65-80 inches

Y is equal to 8.0 if girth is over 80 inches. (One seer is equal to 0.93 kg)

Mullick's formula for Buffaloes

X = 25.156 (Y) - 360.232

X = Estimate of body weight in pounds

Y = Heart girth in inches

Formula of Bandari and team

For dry and non-pregnant buffaloes

Body weight in lbs = -2123.73 + 26.356 (Girth in inches) + 21.50 (Length in inches)

For dry pregnant buffaloes

Body weight in lbs = -1934.48 + 20.52 (Girth in inches) + 25.90 (Length in inches)

For Lactating buffaloes

Body weight in lbs = -2387.60 + 27.12 (Girth in inches) + 24.55 (Length in inches)

2. By weigh band

This is meant for cattle and pigs. It is a printed tape having weights in pounds (lbs) along its border. It is put around the chest and the weight is read directly from the tape. There are three different weights that could be recorded by this band.

1. For lean animal
2. For normal animal and
3. For very fat animal.

Precautions

1. Body measurements should be recorded only when animal is standing calmly and squarely on its feet.
2. Record the observations in the morning.
3. When estimating the weight for medication or to calculate nutrient requirement add 5 per cent additional allowance

Assignment

1. Record the observations on dentition to estimate the age and find the magnitude of difference between estimated and actual age.
2. Record the heart girth, body length of different species and estimate the weight with given formulae. Then find out the magnitude of difference between estimated and actual weight.

Questions

1. Define crown, fang, broken mouth and diastema.
2. Draw the diagram of teeth and label it.

Signature of Teacher

❑❑❑

7

Preparation of Animals for Shows or Judging

Date:

Objective

a) To exhibit the best type of animal and win the cattle show.
b) The individual breeder can exchange ideas & experience in shows.
c) Shows give opportunity for comparison among superior type of animals within and between breeds.
d) Helps new breeders to make contacts with established breeders.
e) Helps in discovering and popularizing better genetic make-up in the various breeds.
f) Increases pride and involvement of the farmers.

Material required

Brushes
Stiff-bristled brushes
Soft-bristled brush
Curry comb
Tail brush or comb

Washing Equipment
Scrub Brush
Hose
Spray nozzle
Soap
Bucket
Cloth to clean ears
Topline brush for the tail

Tack
Nylon halter
Leather show halter
Two-way ties
Neck chains

Feed Supplies
Grain
Hay
Water bucket
Feed tub
Feed scoop

Bedding Supplies
Straw

Clipping Equipment
Large clippers
Small clippers with fine blades
2 sets of blades
Blow dryer
Topline brush
Shavings
Broom
Pitch fork
Shovel

Procedure

Selection of animal

A good animal does not guarantee success in the showring; but without a good animal, it is difficult to consistently do well. Select animal of best-type possessing true breed characteristic *i.e.,* dairy conformation, good temperament, proper growth & development, at least before two month of show. The following points should be considered in selecting an animal for show:

a) The animal needs to be long, stretchy, and of good size for her age and breed.
b) It should have sharp, clean withers, a straight, strong back; a long, level, wide rump; and feet and legs with correct set.
c) The heifer needs to show promise of outstanding udder development and have well-placed teats that hang plumb.
d) It should have a good spring of rib and be deep in the chest and rear flank.
e) The animal needs to be the offspring of a proven bull with high Predicted Transmitting Ability milk and type and out of a cow possessing good type with above-average production.

Feeding the Show Animal

The nutritional needs of your show animal are of major importance. A good balanced ration, built around high-quality forage be given to animal throughout the year. Good forage and hay helps in rumen development,which shows up on the animal as a deep body with a good spring of rib. Animal be fed as so she will be thrifty and dairy-like at show time-not too thin and not too fat. Heifer's body condition can be controlled by the amount of grain fed.Good, fitting rations are light and not too high in protein.

Before taking animal to the show, teach her to eat and drink from the same pails that be used at the show. Animal must have plenty of clean water available at all times.

Trimming Feet of Show Animals

Properly trimmed feet are important and be done two weeks before the show. If the toes are long and unshapely, trim them early in the conditioning period. Heifers with long toes tend to walk on the backs of their heels, detracting from the appearance of the legs.The feet of calves and heifers are much easier to trim than a cow's feet, because they are easier to restrain and the hoof is softer. The toes can be trimmed with hoof nippers. Trimming feet of mature cows can be done by use a sharp, 1-inch woodchisel as the animal stands on a 2-inch-thick board.Experienced trimmers attempt to remove excess toe and sole growth to get the cow forward on her toes and to reduce heel compression. A balanced hoof is important.It is important to avoid making the hoof bleed. If this does happen, the animal may limp for a few days. This is why you need to trim at least 2 weeks before show date.

Clipping Show Animals

Clipping is one of the most important things as it improves the animal's style and overall appearance. Clip animals at least 60 days before the showto allow a new coat to grow back. Most animals do not appreciate clipping. It may be necessary to use a nose lead to pull their heads to a post to prevent them from hitting you when swinging their heads.

Guidelines

- Clip the head, neck, ears, tail, and udder (cows and springing heifers only).
- Clip the front and rear legs so as to have the appearance of greater flatness of bone and to remove stains.
- Trim toplines to improve straightness.
- Clip the withers to a sharp point to improve angularity.
- Body clipping is acceptable, especially when the body hair is excessively long. Do not clip the belly and udder of heifers that have not calved and are not springing.

- Clip the entire head and neck as short as possible. Leave the whiskers on the nose because this makes the muzzle appear wider.
- Clip the inside and outside of the ears. Blend the neck and shoulders by clipping in the direction the hair runs. Start at the point of shoulder, and clip upward to the top of the shoulder blade.

  The arrows on this diagram show the direction you should clip the hair to go against the grain of the hair. The dark grey area along the back is considered the "topline." The light grey areas on the ears and tail show where shorter blade small clippers should be used.

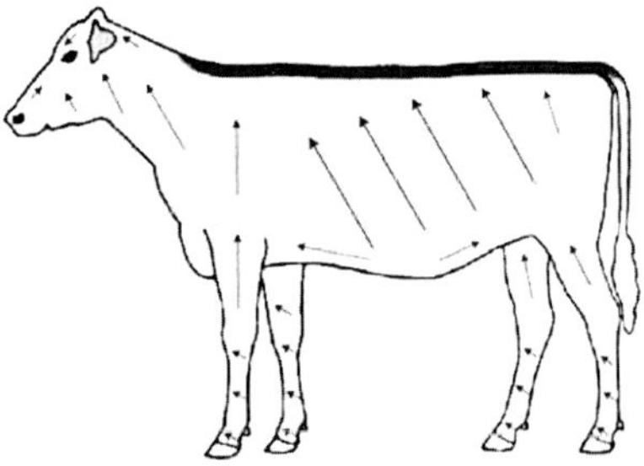

- Use the clippers to make the point of withers as sharp as possible.
- Clip the tail from a point about 4 inches above the hairs on the switch. Clip against the hair on the tail until you reach the tailhead. Blend the longer hair and close-clipped area at the point where the tail lies over the pinbones.
- Don't clip all the hair off the topline. If the topline is not level, clip the high areas and blend these into the lower sections of the topline.
- Every clipping rule recommended for a heifer can be applied to a milking animal. Animals that have freshened will need additional clipping. Clip the udder as close as possible, then clip along the milk veins to make them more noticeable.
- Clip the belly area between the milk veins. Blend all clipper marks, using the natural body lines to help hide them. It is easier to clip a full udder, and you are less apt to cut the skin with the clippers when the udder is full.

Washing Animals

After your animals arrive at the show site, wash them thoroughly. Liquid detergents for kitchen or laundry use are suitable for washing. Use a stiff brush, and work loose all of the dirt next to the hide. When washing around the head, hold the ears closed to prevent water from getting in. Wipe the ears clean with a cloth dampened with rubbing alcohol to remove the ear wax and dirt. Don't forget to wash between the rear legs and udder, an area easily missed. Thoroughly wash the switch; you can remove tangles by using hair conditioner after washing. Animals may have to be spot washed just before the show. Be careful to allow enough time for the animal to dry completely before show time.

Training Animals to Lead and Pose

- It is best to begin with a rope halter for tying the animal in a well-bedded place, but do not lead much in the first couple of days.
- Trainer can begin to teach your show animal to lead by leading it to water twice daily. Within a few days you may begin to take it out for short periods of time.
- After the animal is broken to lead, train it to walk and pose properly. Use a dairy show halter with a chain for this exercise. Train the animal to walk slowly and with short steps with its head carried high.
- Always lead your animal at a normal pace in a clockwise manner; this puts you on the outside of the circle.
- Trainer should walk opposite the head on the left side, holding the lead strap with the right hand close to the halter and the strap neatly, but naturally (preferably not coiled), gathered in one or both hands.
- As the judge studies animal, the preferred method of leading is walking slowly backward, facing the animal and holding the lead strap in the left hand with the extra lead neatly but naturally gathered in one or both hands.
- When given the signal to pull into line, move quickly to that position in the ring. Lead at a comfortable pace with the animal's head held high enough for impressive style, attractive carriage, and graceful walk. Never allow a large gap to occur between your animal and the one ahead of you.
- When posing and showing a dairy animal, stay on the animal's left side and stand faced at an angle to her in a position far enough

away to see the stance of her feet and topline. Pose the animal with her feet squarely placed. The hind leg nearest the judge is to be posed slightly behind the other when showing heifers.

- Do not overshow an animal. When the judge is observing the animal, get the feet posed reasonably well, and let her stand. Do not delay the show inan attempt to pose the feet perfectly.

Assignments

Describe in detail about different preparations of animal before sending her to show.

Questions

1. How soon before the show should you trim the animal feet?
2. How long before the show should you shear a show wether?
3. Name three desirable physical characteristics in heifers for show

What kind of halter can be used when showing?

Signature of Teacher

❑❑❑

8

Selection and Culling of Dairy Animals

Date:

Objective

- To know criteria and characteristics of good dairy animal.
- To judging dairy animals.
- To know the criteria for culling a dairy animal.

Material required

Ready reckoners for ageing, weighing balance, measuring tape, and animals.

Procedure

Selection of Animals

Proper selection of animals for milk yield, fat and protein yield, body capacity and "dairyness" is the first and the most important step to be adopted in successful dairying. Knowledge of the characteristics of good type in dairy cattle is of importance not only to the buyer of new female stock but also to the herd owner who wishes to raise the heifer calves from his best cows to replace cows no longer useful or profitable.

General selection procedures for dairy breeds

Selection of dairy cows

Knowledge of breed standards: Dairy breeds differ in type and characteristics. For example, of the five major exotic breeds of dairy cattle, the Jersey excels in symmetry and development of the udder. The Guernsey cow possesses desired characteristics such as good dairy tendency and angularity. These qualities are somewhat less pronounced, however, than in the Jersey breed. Selection of a proper dairy animal partly depends on familiarity with the standards and ideals of the breed.

The distinguishing features of the dairy type of cow, as seen in a good dairy cow are:

1. Angularity of form, 2. Development of milking organs, 3. Development of feeding capacity.

Angularity of form

After calving, a good dairy cow loses weight and becomes angular in appearance. This means that parts of the skeleton, such as the withers, shoulders, backbone, hips, and pin bones, project more from the body and appear to be much sharper. The dairy-cattle breeds differ in their angularity and there are also great differences between cows of the same breed in this characteristic, though the best dairy cows are, as a rule, the most angular. Viewed from the side, a cow with a deep, long body with wide, well-sprung ribs is said to have a large body capacity. Angularity must be considered with the degree of fleshiness. Cows differ greatly in the amounts of flesh that they carry and good dairy cows usually put on fat and gain in weight during the dry period.

Development of milking organs

A high-producing cow requires a capacious udder.The udder must be soft, pliable, silky in texture and sack-like in nature. Ideally, the udder, should not hang below the cow's hock when viewed from the side. Nature of attachment of udder through central, or median, suspensory ligaments are very important. This must be extremely strong and well attached. It is an accepted fact that an udder with an excellent central ligament is a long-lasting one.

Teat placement is next in importance. Ideally, the front teats should be even and centrally placed on each quarter of the udder. Teat size (over- and undersized teats should be avoided), shape and placement are highly heritable.

The udders of greatest capacity have a high proportion of secreting tissue and they collapse, or reduce greatly in size, following milking. Udders with relatively small proportions of secreting tissue and higher amount of connective tissue do not show so much reduction in size with milking and have a firmer consistency.

Development of feeding capacity

Large body capacity is associated with ample space for the rumen and digestive system, and this, in turn, is associated with superior milk production. The barrel includes all the middle portion of the animal extending from the backbone to the under line and from the shoulders and chest to hip bone and flank, or it may be said to include all the region between the fore legs and rear legs except the udder. Capacity of barrel depends upon the depth of the barrel from top to bottom and also on its width, or the distance through the barrel in a horizontal direction at right angles to the backbone.

Dairyness: High-producing dairy cows have a strong stimulus to convert the nutrients in their feed into milk rather than into body muscle or fat (beef type).Most cows that have a strong stimulus for milk production have an angular form, with no more flesh than is necessary for good health and condition, extraordinary development of milking organs, and large feeding capacity in proportion to body size. It is this external evidence of productive ability, or dairy tendency, that is most often relied upon in selecting dairy cows. As previously stated, the most reliable guide to a cow's productive ability is a record of her milk and butterfat yields, but such a record is often not available.

Summary of Characteristics indicating ideal dairy animal

A. **Body form**

Desirable features: A well-balanced proportionate body parts.Evidence of the three distinguishing features of dairy type: angularity of form, development of milking organs, and development of feeding capacity.

Undesirable features: Lack of angularity; poorly developed milking organs or feeding capacity; parts poorly proportioned.

B. **Dairy tendency**

Desirable features: Prominent points of the body plainly visible, thighs relatively thin and wide apart to make room for udder.

Undesirable features: Blocky form with thick covering of fatty tissue. Heavy thighs, legs set close together.

C. **Size**

Desirable features: Large and well grown for age, without roughness and coarseness, breed considered. Large cows have greater producing capacity than small cows. Weightage be for the respective breeds.

Undesirable features: Undersized for age or distinctly stunted.

D. **Rump**

Desirable features: Good length and breadth; level; evident capacity for giving birth to calf; freedom from roughness and coarseness; smooth, level top line. Cows with broad, level rumps are said to have more capacious udders than those with sloping rumps.

Undesirable features: Rump sloping toward the rear as a result of the pin bones being lower than the hip bones; sloping forward; or sloping to the side from the top line toward the thurls. Rump short and narrow at the hip bones or pin bones.

E. **Style and activity**

Desirable features: Head held up strongly and the top line of the back nearly straight. Strong, straight legs placed squarely under the body and a good carriage with regular and even gait. Docile but active and alert disposition, as shown by bright, prominent eyes and tendency to observe activities about her. All parts well-proportioned and no marked defects.

Undesirable features: Dull, deep-set eyes; easily frightened and untractable. Rough, uneven top line. A sway-backed top line detracts from the appearance of the animal but does not necessarily indicate physical weakness. Sway-backed condition. Legs crooked as viewed from the side or rear; rear feet and legs turned outward; uneven gait; crooked neck, or ewe-neck; lameness; winged shoulders.

CULLING OF DAIRY ANIMALS

Culling is elimination of non-productive, uneconomic, diseased and undesirable animals from the herd.Well-planned culling strategies can improve the bottom line, in times and significantly impact dairy herd profitability.

Reasons for Culling

There are many reasons to cull cattle. Dairy farmers are focused on maximising income while at the same time controlling all production costs. One area which merits considerable attention, but is all too often is ignored, is the cost of maintaining the herd size, a major driver of turnover. Culling rates in the organized herd of India range from 20-25% on average but may go to well over 35% per annum, where more management control could be applied. Among many reasons for culling dairy cows, common are: underproductive, uneconomic, poor production, or very poor reproductive ability, with sterility problems and breeding, irregularities, very poor conditions, stunted growth, suffering from incurable illness, or disease animals found to be positive for serious infectious diseases like Tuberculosis, Johnes disease, Brucellosis, loss of one or more quarters and teats of the udder due to chronic mastitis resulting in marked reduction in milk production.

Culling dairy animals: Decision checklist

1. Milk production 20 percent below the herd average.
2. Chronic mastitis case.
3. Long Dry period (four months or more).
4. Hard milker. Difficult to milk the animal due to udder shape or teat structure.
5. History of calving difficulties or post calving illnesses such as retained placenta, metritis, or milk fever.
6. Timid cow or nervous cow or kicking whenever udder is touched.
7. Old cow (pariety>8) and needed to be replaced with freshening heifers.
8. Cow with a long calving interval.

Questions

1. Discuss in detail the criteria to be considered while selecting good dairy type animal.
2. Define culling. What criteria would you consider while culling an animal?

Signature of Teacher

❑❑❑

9

Preparation of Project Report for Establishment of Small-scale Dairy Unit

Date:

Objective

- To know different components of economics of dairy farming.
- To prepare a project report for establishing small-scale dairy unit

Material required

Calculator, notebook

Procedure

India has recently made amazing development in strengthening the dairy sector. From anonymity in the field of major milk producers in the world not very long ago, our country has reached the top position as the highest milk producer, recently bypassing the USA. As per FAO estimate, India now has the largest number of cattle, 190.90 millions and 108.70 millions buffaloes, which accounts for respectively 16% and 53% of the total world population. Annual milk production now stands at 142 million metric tonnes (2014-15).

In this scenario we can understand feasibility and cost & return involved in a 10 unit buffalo farm by following assumptions:

1. The breeds are graded Murrah buffaloes. Freshly calved Murrah female buffaloes in 1st or 2nd lactation will be purchased in two batches of five animals each/batch at an interval of 5 to 6 months.
2. Lactation and dry periods are 270 and 90 days, respectively.
3. The markets are considered for both inputs and outputs.
4. Availability of 02 acres of land for fodder cultivation is prerequisite for the project.

5. Cost of rearing calves not considered as it will be repealed by their sale.
6. Heifers will be used as replacement stocks.

Parameters for estimating feasibility of the project

Parameters used for the economic analysis of the feasibility of the project are Net Present Values (NPV), Benefit Cost Ratio (B.C. Ratio) and payback period. In all methods, a minimum acceptable discount rate is specified to consider the time value of money.

NPV = Discount net returns - Initial investment.

The formula for NPV is: $NPV = \frac{B_0 - C_0}{(1+i)^0} + \frac{B_1 - C_1}{(1+i)^1} + ... + \frac{Br - Cr}{(1+i)^r}$

Where: t = year, B = benefits, C = cost, i=discounted cash flow rate.

The project will be viable if NPV is greater than 0

B:C Ratio = Discounted net returns/Initial investments.

The project will be acceptable if these are more than unity.

Payback period is the time period in which the project will return sufficient money to cover the initial investment.

Techno economic parameters

S.No.	Parameters	Value
1.	Cost of Animal (Rs./animal) including transportation	60000
2.	Average Milk Yield (litre/day)	12
3.	Covered Floor space per adult animal(sq.ft)	30
4.	Open space per adult animal(sq.ft)	100
5.	Manger length/animal in inches	25
6.	Covered Floor space per young stock (sq.ft)	15
7.	Open space per young stock (sq.ft)	50
8.	Manger per young stock in inches	15
9.	Construction cost of office & store in sq.ft	250
10.	Cost of construction per sq.ft (Rs) for covered space	200
11.	Cost of other equipment per animal (Rs.)	1000
12.	Cost of fodder cultivation (Rs./acre/season)	5000

13.	Insurance premium (% per annum)	5
14.	Veterinary aid/animal/ year (Rs.)	1000
15.	Cost of concentrate feed (Rs./kg)	16
16.	Cost of dry fodder (Rs./kg)	2
17.	Rate of interest (%)	12
18.	Repayment period (years)	6
19.	Selling price of milk/litre (Rs./kg)	30
20.	Sale price of gunny bags (Rs. per bag)	10
21.	Lactation days	270
22.	Dry days	90

Calculation of Feed requirement and cost of feed per animal per day

FEEDING STUFF	**COST/KG**	**lactation period**		**dry period**	
	Rs.	**Qty (kg)**	**Cost (Rs.)**	**Qty (kg)**	**Cost (Rs.)**
Concentrate feed	16	7kg	112	2	32
Green fodder	1	25	farm grown	20	farm grown
Dry fodder	2	6	12	5	10
Total	124	42			

Calculation of days-in-milk and dry days

Lactation chart/Dry chart						
Animal	Year I	Year II	Year III	Year IV	Year V	Year VI
Batch I	* **					
Batch II						
Days-in-milk	2250	2700	2700	2700	2700	2700
Dry Days	1350	900	900	900	900	900

Each batch consists of five buffaloes

* Shaded blocks indicates days-in-milk; one block = 90days

** Empty block indicates dry days; one block = 90 days

Calculation of Feed cost

Particulars	Years					
	I	II	III	IV	V	VI
Lactation Days	279000	334800	334800	334800	334800	334800
Dry Days	56700	37800	37800	37800	37800	37800
Total	335700	372600	372600	372600	372600	372600

Estimation of Project cost and bank loan (Cost. In Rs.)

Components	Cost. In Rs.
A) Capital cost	
Covered area for 10 buffaloes @ 30sq.ft/buffalo@200/sqft	60000
Covered area 10 calves 15 sq.ft./calf @200/sq.ft.	30000
Cost of construction of boundary & manger for open space for adult & calves	70000
Cost of construction store room 60 sq.ft @300 per sq.ft	18000
Cost of construction of office cum marketing room 100 sq ft @400 per sq.ft	40000
Cost of 10 Murrah buffaloes @60000/buffaloes including transportation	600000
Cost of dairy appliance @Rs.1000/Buffalo	10000
Electrification	6000
Total	834000
B) Recurring cost to be capitalized	
Cost of feed for first batch of 5 buffaloes for one month	18600
Cost of insurance 5 animals @5% of animal cost	15000
Cost of fodder cultivation in 2 acres of land/year	10000
Cost of medicine vaccine, electricity for the first month	2000
Contingency	10000
Total recurring expenditure	55600
TOTAL PROJECT COST	889600
Margin money 25% of project cost	222400
Loan Amount	667200

Calculation of Loan amount and repayment schedule

Loan amount = 667200; grace period= 6 months

Loan amount at the end of grace period=667200+40032=707232

Amortization Table - Yearly View

Year	Starting Balance	Interest Paid	Principle Paid	Repayment (Yearly)	Ending Balance
I	707232	80258.07	85660.17	165918.24	621571.83
II	621571.83	74644.7	105100.06	165918.24	525047.81
III	525047.81	56064.91	109853.33	165918.24	416282.14
IV	416282.14	42132.76	123785.52	165918.28	293722.23
V	293722.23	26433.65	139484.64	165918.29	155618.61
VI	155618.61	8743.51	143348.28	165918.29	0.00
TOTAL PAYMENT		288277.6	707232	995509.6	

Calculation of Annual Depreciation cost

Item	Initial Cost	Depreciation cost/Year					
		I	II	III	IV	V	VI
Buildings	218000	0	21800	19620	17658	15892	14303
Animal	600000	0	60000	54000	48600	43740	39366
Equipments	60000	0	6000	5400	4860	4374	3937
Total	-	**0**	**87800**	**79020**	**71118**	**64006**	**57606**

Calculation of annual recurring cost

Cost component	Year					
	I	II	III	IV	V	VI
Repayment of loan	165919	165919	165919	165919	165919	165919
Feed costs	335700	372600	372600	372600	372600	372600
Insurance Premium	26500	30000	30000	30000	30000	30000
Depreciation cost	0	87800	79020	71118	64006	57606
Medicine, Electricity	7500	10000	10000	10000	10000	10000
Fodder cultivation	10000	10000	10000	10000	10000	10000
Total Costs	**545619**	**676319**	**667539**	**659637**	**652525**	**646125**

Income

Component	Year					
	I	II	III	IV	V	VI
Sale of milk	1012500	1215000	1215000	1215000	1215000	1215000
Sale of gunny bag	2500	2700	2700	2700	2700	2700
Gross return	1015000	1217700	1217700	1217700	1217700	1217700

Calculation of BCR

Component	Year					
	I	II	III	IV	V	VI
Capital Costs	834000	0	0	0	0	0
Recurring Cost	545619	676319	667539	659637	652525	646125
Total Costs	1379619	676319	667539	659637	652525	646125
Gross return	1015000	1217700	1217700	1217700	1217700	1217700
Net Benefit	-364619	541381	550161	558063	565175	571575
Discount Factor* @15% discounted cash flow (DF)	1.00	1.15	1.32	1.52	1.75	2.01
Present Worth Benefit	1015000	1058870	920756	800658	696224	605412
Present Worth Cost	1379619	588103	504755	433722	373083	321238

* Calculated as $(1+r)^t$; where, r=0.15; t = respective year

Financial indicators of Project Viability

S.No	Financial indicators	Estimated value	Preferred value
1.	PW costs @ 15%DF	3600521	
2.	PW benefits @ 15%DF	5096919	
3.	Net Present Value (NPV)	1496398	Should be +ve
4.	Benefit Cost Ratio (BCR)	1.42:1	>1

Feasibility analysis

Thus from above analysis it is found that NPV is Rs. 1496398, which is greater than zero. Also Benefit Cost Ratio is found out to be 1.42, which is more than unity.

Thus, from all the aspects the feasibility analysis one can say the project is viable one.

Assignments

Prepare a project report for establishing 50 cow unit with feasibility analysis.

Questions

1. What is Net Present Value?
2. How to calculate B:C ratio?

Signature of Teacher

❑❑❑

UNIT-II

Introduction

Date:

Livestock rearing is one of the foremost occupations in India besides as a source of food. It also provides manure, draught power for agriculture and local transportation. Significance of the livestock sector can be appreciated from the fact that it contributes about 8.5-9% to the country's GDP. From this it is clearthat the contribution to the GDP fromlivestock sector istoo low for such a large size of livestock population. The reason oflow productivity from thissector isattributable to underfeeding of the livestock. An idea of the meager fodder availability can be had from the fact that about 50% of the cattle population, depending largely upon free rangeland grazing in forests, pastures, village commons and the like, end up getting only about 1.5 kg of dry fodder/ day/ ACU (Adult Cattle Unit) as against the healthy fodder requirement norm of 3% body weight (Planning commission of India,2011) Thusincreasing cattle population by animal husbandry policies, without giving attention towards enhancing the forage production, is possibly put further pressure on the already meager fodder resources in the country and thus causing further depletion in productivity of this sector.

Major Fodder Sources in India and their Status (Planning commission of India, 2011)

A. **Tropical and Sub-tropical Grasslands:** These are mid-successional/sub-climax type of Grasslands and are found in high rainfall areas (western ghats) to arid/semi-arid areas including Terai and Gangetic plains,they are prone to periodic burning and are subjected to heavy grazing. So this has resulted in their general degradation and very low productivity. Such type of grasslands form important source of fodder for the livestock maintained by poor and landless people.

B. **Shola Grasslands:** These are Climatic climax type of grassland and this climax stage is maintained by severe frost and recurrent fires. The major intervention in Shola grasslands is on account of attempts to bring these under tree plantations.

C. **Alpine, Sub-alpine Meadows:** These are Climatic climax type of pastures and during summers usually witness the intensive transhumant grazing activity. The climax stage is maintained by severe winters, high velocity winds and frost. The alpine and sub-alpine meadows are suffering from general degradation, increasing incidence of non-palatable species and erosion due to overgrazing.

D. **Village Commons, Fallows & Wastelands:** The forages from these lands are important source of feed to the village cattle. But now, most of these lands have been diverted for other uses, and whatever is remaining has become badly fragmented and degraded with no management concerns.

E. **Forests:** Forests of almost all crown density classifications, and the natural blanks contained within these, form an important source of forage. However, free grazing and invasion by exotic weeds has resulted in degradation of the ground cover of fodder value in the forests.

F. **Tree-leaf fodder:** Tree leaf fodder is a very important source of forage, especially during pinch periods. Less prone to periodic droughts, trees form an assured source of fodder year after year. The major sources of tree leaf fodder are the trees growing on forests and common lands.However, with high timber value plantations coming up on scrub forests, this resource is getting depleted from near habitations. Another source of tree leaf fodder is the trees growing on farm lands. However, with traditional cropping practices giving way to intensive agriculture, thissource of tree leaf fodder is getting depleted.

G. **Cultivated Fodder & Crop Residue:** Meets about half of fodder requirement in the country. However, its availability is limited to the arable lands and land rich farmers.

Table: Percent contribution of different fodder sources in India

Sources	Quantity
Crop Residues	54%
Cultivated fodder	28%
Grasslands	18%

Source: Hegde (2006)

Table 1revealed that both dry and green fodder availability of has not been matching with the requirement. Also by 2020the projected shortage of green fodder is more than 60%and in dry fodder the value is near to 23%.

Fodder Availability – Demand and Supply Status:
Country scenario

Table-2. Demand and Supply Status of Fodder Resources in India (in Million Ton)	Supply		Demand		Shortfall	
	Green	Dry	Green	Dry	Green	Dry
2000	384.5	428	988	549	604	121
2005	389.9	443	1025	569	635	126
2010	395.2	451	1061	589	666	138
2015	400.6	466	1097	609	696	143
2020	405.9	473	1134	630	728	157

Source: Draft Report of the WG on Animal Husbanry and Dairying for 5-year Plan (2002-2007). Planning Commissoion of India, August 2001.

State scenario

Broad picture of region-wise availability offodder in J& K state(lakh MT on DM basis)

Land Resources	Region			Total
	Jammu	Kashmir	Ladakh	
1. From uncultivated land				
i) Forests (village papers)	9.79	0.078	0.0009	9.87
ii) Barren and uncultivated land	2.29	0.29	0.298	2.88
iii) Non-agricultural land	2.29	0.56	0.040	2.88
iv) Cultivable waste land	1.03	0.50	0.11	2.25
v) Permanent pastures	2.49	1.33	0.032	3.85
vi) Land under tree groups	0.28	0.05	0.008	0.34
Total	18.76	2.82	0.49	22.06
2. From uncultivated private support land				
i) Fallow land	0.75	1.01	0.014	1.77
ii) Orchards	0.028	0.84	0.008	0.87
iii) Fodder from bunds and paddy field	0.29	0.35	0.00	0.64
Total	1.07	2.20	0.022	3.29
3. Cultivated land under food/ forage/other crops				
Fodder crops	1.86	0.71	0.16	2.74

Region-wise requirement and availability of fodder (lakh M.T on DM Basis) in J&Kfrom all sources

S.No.	Region	Requirement	Availability	% deficiency
1.	Jammu	100.08	54.10	45.94
2.	Kashmir	43.95	20.06	54.35
3.	Ladakh	4.68	1.43	69.44
	Overall	148.17	75.59	49.17

Fodder as a source of energy and nutrients supply

All animalsneedenergy to facilitate them to live and reproduce and the only source to getenergy is the feed they eat.Thus all animalsdirectly or indirectly are dependent on theplants. Plantsgive energythrough organic compounds like proteins, carbohydrates and fats. Besides these, plants also contain minerals, vitamins and water. Thus breakdown of feed originated from plants to different components in animalsis like that

Classification of feed and fodders

A. **Roughages**: These are feed stuffs which contain more than 18 percent crude fiber (cellulose, hemi-cellulose and lignin) and less than 60 percent Total Digestible Nutrients. Further they are of two types:

1. Green or succulent roughages - These roughageshaveabout 60-90 percent moisture e.g pastures, cultivated fodders, tree leaves, root crops and silages.
2. Dry roughages - These roughages contain about 10-15 percent moisture e.g. Straw and Hay

B. **Concentrates**: They are concentrated source of nutrients and therefore, they have higher nutritive value and energythan roughagesthey contain less than 18 percent crude fibre and more than 60 percent TDN. They are less bulky and have higher digestibility. Furtherconcentrates areclassified as:

1. Energy Rich Concentrates - e.g. Cereal grains, cereal grain by-products, Roots and tubers.
2. Protein Rich Concentrates - i) Plant origin e.g. Oilseed cake, pulse chuni, Brewer's grains and yeast. ii) Animal origin e.g. Fish meal, Meat meal, Blood meal.

C. **Feed supplements** are those compoundswhich are used to improve the nutritional value of the basal feeds so as to take care of any deficiency, e.g.

1. Vitamin supplements
2. Mineral supplements

D. **Feed Additives**

These areadded in small quantity for the fortification to basal feed in order to improve feed efficiency and productive performance of the animals. Some commonly used feed additives are as below:

1. Antibiotics
2. Enzymes

6. Bio stimulators
7. Antioxidants

3. Hormones
4. Thyroprotein
5. Probiotics
8. Mold inhibitors
9. Pellet binders
10. Coccidiostats

Significance of Fodder

- Fodder plants supplement the quality nutritional requirements for the animal body. Eg.Berseem, Cowpea, Lucerne etc.
- Fodder plantation increase the potential carrying capacity of a given farm and thus animals have not toexert excessive grazing pressure on the farmlands and pastures.
- More animals are kept in a lesser space when supplemented with fodder as compared to when they graze on the same rangeland full time.
- Feed cost is reduced due to more fodder plantations and thus there is gain in profits over the time.
- Excess fodders can be stored and preserved as silage and hay which can be used for the lean period when there is fodder scarcity.
- Growing leguminous fodders increase nutritional status of the land further soil erosion is reduced.
- Sick animals which are under treatment can be fed on fodders and also with the help of these crops the young ones adapt to grazing smoothly.

❑❑❑

10

Visit to the Fodder Farm

Date:

Objectives

- To get acquainted with the Fodder farm of and physical facilities available.
- To get familiarize with different fodder crops being raised at farm.
- To get first hand information regarding management practices followed.

Material required

- Notebook
- Pen/pencil
- Apron

Procedure

The students along with the course instructor will visit the fodder farmto get acquainted withscientific management operations being adopted to manage the fodder farm.

Observations

The following observations should be recorded during visit:

1. Area offarm
2. Manpower involved at farm
3. No. of fodder crops being maintained
4. Details of fodder crops being maintained at farm

5. Method of sowing adopted for fodder crop
6. Type offertilisers being used at farm
7. Source of irrigation and number of irrigations
8. Any other information.

Precautions

- Do not damage the crop at fodder farm
- Watch undergoing activities carefully.

Questions

1. Why is it important to know about the fodder crops?
2. What is the importance of fodder crops?

Signature of Teacher

❏❏❏

11

Familiarization with the Various Types of Fodder in the State and India

Date:

Objectives

- To get familiarize with the various types of fodder crops utilized in the state and samples of fodder in India
- To know theclassification ofdifferentfodder crops for their proper management.

Material Required

- Fodder crops
- Chart, photograph etc. offodder crops

Procedure

The students along with the course instructor will visit the fodder farm to discuss the various aspects of fodder crops i.e identification of different fodder crops,their classification and management practices.

Classification of fodder crops

1. Kharif

a) Annual

- Leguminous (cowpea, clusterbean)
- Non-leguminous (sorghum, maize, teosinite, bajra, jowar, pioneer jowar)
- Grasses (Deenanath, Kazungala)

b) Perennial

- Leguminous (Lucern)
- Non-leguminous (Hybrid napier)

2. Rabi

a) Annual

- Leguminous (Berseem)
- Non-leguminous (oats)

b) Perennial

- Leguminous (Lucern)

3. Zaid (April-June)

- Leguminous (Cowpea, field bean, guar)
- Non-leguminous (maize, M.P. charri, Bajra etc.)

4. On the basis of nutrient density in the dry matter

a) Roughages

- Non-maintenance (Wheat straw, paddy straw,maize stover etc.)
- Maintenance (Jowar, Bajra, N.B.-21)
- Productive (**Low protein:** oat, Maize, Barley, Charri; **High Protein** : Berseem, Lucerne, Cowpea etc.)

b) Concentrates

- Carbonaceous (rich in energy, low in DCP, cereal grains)
- Proteinous (rich in DCP, ground nut cake, til and mustard cake)
- Agro-industrialby-products
- Animal products (Fish meal, frog meal and meatmeal)

5. On the basis of plant-type

- Cultivated
- Pastures

- Forest edible
- Plantation
- Aquatic

Observation

- Name the fodder and their identification characteristics

Activities

1. Prepare a herbarium forgreen fodder crops utilized in the state and their seed collection.
2. Name the varieties of different fodder crops usedin India.

Questions

1. What is the growing season ofkharif and rabi fodders?

Signature of Teacher

❐❐❐

12

Familiarization with the Various Fertilizers and Manures

Date:

Objectives

- To get acquainted with different fertilizers use to grow fodder crop.
- To get familiarize with different manures use in fodder crops.

Material required

Different fertilizers and manures to identify

Procedure

Different synthetic fertilizers and manures are shown to the students.

Plant Nutrition The nutritional needs of plants can be catagorised in to :

1. **Primary macro nutrients**: These are six nutrients needed by plants in large quantities.viz. Carbon (C), Hydrogen (H), Oxygen (O), Nitrogen (N), Phosphorus (P) and Potassium (K).
2. **Secondary macro nutrients**: These are nutrients needed byplants in significant quantities viz. Calcium (Ca), Sulfur (S) and Magnesium (Mg).
3. **Micro nutrients**: These are seven nutrients needed by plants in small quantities viz. Iron (Fe), Molybdenum (Mo), Boron (B), Copper (Cu), Manganese (Mn), Zinc (Zn) and Chlorine (Cl).
4. **Miscellaneous:** These nutrients may also be required in some plant varieties in small quantities viz. Silicon (Si), Cobalt (Co), Selenium (Se), Sodium (Na), Vanadium (V) and Chlorine.

Classification of fertilizers

1. Organic manures

a) Bulky organic manures
- Farm yard manure
- Compost
- Vermicompost
- Green manure

b) Concentrated organic manures
- Edible oil cakes
- Non-edible oil cakes
- Blood meal
- Fish meal
- Bone meal

2. Chemical fertilizers

a) Simple fertilizer(Straight fertilizer contain single nutrient)
- Nitrogenous (Urea 46%N)
- Phosphorus (DAP 16% N and 46% P_2O_5)
- Potassium (Muriate of potash 60% K_2O)

b) Complex fertilizer (Multi-nutrient fertilizer contain more than two nutrients)

c) Soil amendments

d) Micro-nutrient mixture

3. Bio fertilizers

- Rhizobium
- Azotobacter
- Azospirillium
- Blue green algae
- Azolla
- Mycorrhizae

Further some fertilizers are **complete** as they contain all the three primary nutrients i.e N,P,K whereas **incomplete** fertilizers donot contain all the three primary nutrients. **Soluble** fertilizers can dissolve in water and use as fertigation whereas **insoluble** fertilisers are granular type and there release is further slow down.

Observations

- Observevarious types of fertilisers. Name them and classify them

Questions

1. What is the difference between organic and inorganic fertilizers?
2. What are thefertilizer source of N,P and K usedfor fodder production?
3. How fertilizer use efficiency can be increased?

Signature of Teacher

❑❑❑

13

Collection, Preservation and Storage of Feed and Fodder; Damages or Loss During Transfer and Storage; Methods to Prevent Them

Date:

Objectives

- To get familiarize with different methods of collecting, preserving and storing of feed and fodder.
- To know the advantage of preserving and storing fodder.

Material Required

- Pictures, charts of different type of preservation and storage methods.

Silage

Scarcity of green forage during lean period can be overcome by storing and preserving the fodders in to silage or hay. Silage is the fermented productformedby the bacteria. These bacteria are present in the air and on the crop andthey producesome acidwhich preserve the nutrient substances in the plant material. This process of making silage is called ensiling.

Crops suitable for silage making

There is a wide choice of crops that are suitable to make silage. Excellent silage can be made from crops like Jowar, Maize, Bajra Oats and Barely which contain high amount of carbohydrates. Among the perennial grasses Hybrid Napier grass, Guinea grass, Para grass, Sudan grass and Rhode grass are used for silage making.

Natural grasses such as *dub, Kolu Katai* could very well be converted into silage instead of allowing them to mature and become less nutritious. Legumes like berseem, lucerne and cowpea are not suitable for silage making. However when mixed with non-legume crops in the right proportion, the mixture yields a well balanced silage. Silage can be made successfully by mixing of paddy straw and berseem, paddy straw and water-hyacinth and berseem and oats.

Stage of harvesting the crop

The fodder crop should be harvested neither immature nor over mature with enough dry matter (30-35%)when there nutrient content is at peak stage having sufficient sugars and carbohydrates. So that the preservative acids i.e. lactic acid is released more.Flowering to milk stage is recommended for making silage from maize, Jowar and oats crops. Whereas boot stage is best in case of bajra and teosinte and in Hybrid napier and Guinea grass 1.25 meter height stage is recommended. For desired dry matter take a handful of chaffed fodder in between the hands and press.If hands do not get moist, the fodder is ready to use for silage.

Ensiling process

There are four methods to produce and store the silage: in a pit, a trench, a tower and for small quantities in sacks. In Jammu preferably the trench silo is recommended with 10m long, 8 m wide and 2m deep for packing of 300-400 quintals of chaffed green fodder. It can supply silage for 10 dairy animals for four months at therate of 20-30 kg per head per day.

Filling the silo

1. Chop the harvested croppack it in to silo trench, fill the trench up to 1m above the ground.
2. Cover it with a layer of 10-15 cm thick of rice straw or wheat bhusa. Cover the straw layer with moist earth and then mud plaster to make the silo trench completely air tight.
3. Keep an occasional watch on it, if there is any crack, plug it immediately.
4. Silage will be ready for feeding after 45 days.

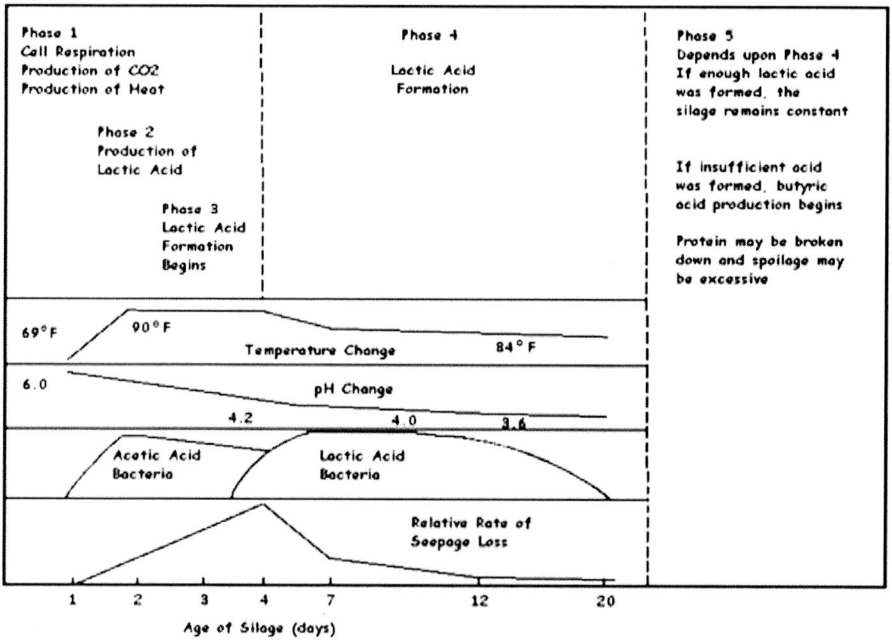

What Happens in the Silo

Graphic Source : Web Resource

Many additives are available to promote fermentation and preservation or inhibit detrimental processes within the silo. Additives that promote lactic acid bacteria are stimulants. Inhibitors slow down undesirable activity. Silage additives are added during wilting or storage. At first molasses were added, then urea to promote lactic acid bacteria growth. More recently bacterial inoculants are used to help natural lactic acid bacteria and lower pH. These additives work best when natural lactic acid bacteria is low as in grass and legume silage. Enzymes are also available to break down forage fiber. Ammonia and acid products are commonly used as well. Dry matter loss can be reduced with the addition of additives but many involve some danger to human health. A firm understanding of the ensiling process is needed for a producer to wisely decide on using additives.

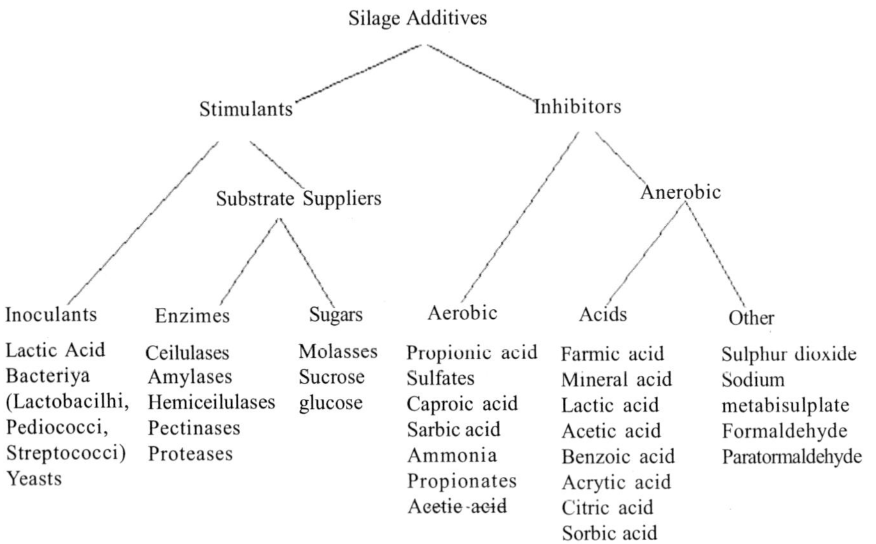

Graphic Source : Web Resource

Feeding the silage

For the first few feedings the animals may dislike its taste.Help them to develop the taste by mixing 5 to 10 kg of silage in their green fodder ration for the first 5 to 6 days.After the taste is developed 20 to 30 kg of silage along with other fodders may be fed per head per day. Silage feeding should be done after milting the milch cattle to avoid the carry over flavor of silage to milk.

Hay making

Hay making is another process to preserve the cut green fodder from rotting and decomposing by drying it in sun and wind and reducing the moisture content from 80 % in the fresh forage to less than 20 %.Hay may be made from legumes, Non-legumes and by mixing both of them.

Curing and storing of hay

Hay should have the dry matter of 82-85% whereas; the fresh forage contains 80-85% moisture. In actual to reduce the respiration losses the hay curing should be completed in short time i.e within 4-5 days. Many factors like crop, weather and management help in hay curing and drying. As per the cop factor the plant species (thin stemmed, grasses and legumes dry quickly), crop maturity stage (In grasses and legumes, the cutting should be done when the first ears appear and blooming starts), initial moisture present in the crops affects it. Weather factors i.e intensity of solar radiation, air temperature, wind speed, relative humidity and soil moisture content affects hay curing and drying. Whereas in management, shattering and turning the crop soon after cutting, when the plants are still green and moist will shorten the drying period. This practice should be done only once, when the plants become dry, they should be touched as little as possible. In case the crop is dried quickly no significance change in aroma and flavour will be observed and the hay remains highly palatable. The cut crop is dried in the sun for approx. 2 days till the moisture is reduced to 15-20 %. This stage is reached when no moisture can be drawn from the stem of the grass when it is pressed with the fingernail. After removing the hay from the field it can bundle in small bundles or boxed and tied. Then it is stored under roof in a shed, so that no rain can enter and deteriorate it.

Effective hay preservatives are used to inhibit microbial growth or artificial drying to remove excess moisture.these include organic acids (propionic and acetic acid), buffer acid and ammoniasources such as anhydrous ammonia and urea.

Losses and damages during collection and preservation of fodder crops

Many different losses typically 20-30% can occur from harvesting and feeding the crop. During ensiling the losses are like respiration, fermentation and effluent are common. The fermentation (actual acid forming process) and respiration losses may be 10 to 15 per cent of dry matter in the original crop, seepage losses may account for about 6 per cent. Excessive aerobic fermentation reduces the energy content of the silage and may cause heat damage to proteins. Less production of acids in foragecause rotting due to more production of undesirable bacteria's that produce enzymes causing an off flavour and slimy silage. Whereas more acid formation by using immature crops having more sugars produce sour and unpalatable silage, when silage contains too much moisture undesirable fermentation takes place the silage will become sour but if the moisture is less the silage will not pack well, air will left and moulds are developed.

Whereas in hay curing and drying mechanical shattering and rain damages are also predominant. Ifit is too wet, losses are likely to occur from heating and mould development.If it is too dry (88%) it is likely to be stalk and dusty. Slow drying during hay making causes loss of feed value.Forage containing more than 40% moisture resist mechanical shattering however as the fodder become drier than 40% moisture, shatter losses increase rapidly. Conventional silage-making reduces field losses as compared to haymaking, but has large capital costs.

Prevention

Good management practices are very important to keep losses at a minimum. It is essential to harvest forage at the best time and then to store it properly to reduce losses. The crops should be cut and ensiled at the same day to avoid the field losses.The moisture content of plants to be ensiled should be about 65%-70%. When the forage to be ensiled is below 30% dry matter, an additive may be needed to reduce the growth of clostridia. Low dry matter content will also produce seepage losses so to soak up theexcess moisture corn cobs, sunflowers, alfala cubes, or even newspaper can be added to the forage. Suitable crop with proper stage and moisture content is another important consideration to reduce the losses. To maintain the quality of the silage in the ensiling process the aerobicphase should be as short as possible. Filling of the silo pits should be done quickly and air should be pushed out with compaction to control fermentation, respiration and heating losses. Next, sealing is another most important operation of any silage making. Breakdown in plastic seal should be controlledtoavoid air entry. Caution should be taken in opening a silo silage should be taken out in section, exposing only a small surface at a time. The exposed portion as far as possible is kept covered.

The best way to reduce loss of hay quality by heating is to ensure that the hay is sufficiently dry before baling. Anything that reduces contact with wet ground, such as old fence posts or free draining gravel, will reduce losses. Good hay is made from high-quality forage cut at the optimum growth stage, then dried and stored as quickly as possible.

Observations

- Enlist the different fodder crops used for silage and hay making.

Activities

1. Make calendar showing green fodder supply round the year

Questions

1. Why should silage trench preferably be located at a place with higher elevation?
2. Explain hay makingunder headings : Sun drying, Barn drying, Dehydration of forages
3. Why a fodder crop that contains a high percentage of carbohydrates is ideal for silage?

Signature of Teacher

❑❑❑

14

Cost Calculation of Fodder Production

Date:

Objectives

- To calculate the cost of cultivation for different fodder crops.
- To get acquainted with different input sources used in the calculation of cost.

Material required

- Cost of inputsused for producing the fodder crops.
- Amount of inputs.

Pre-requisite

- Time consumed in the preparation of land.
- Seed rate of different fodder crops.
- Nutritional requirements ofdifferent fodder crops.
- Number of mandays involved for growing different fodder crops.

Procedure

Cost of calculation of berseem fodder production

S.No.	Input	Quantity/ ha	Unit	Rate (Rs)	Amount (Rs)
1	Land preparation	2.5	Hr	500	1250
2	Puddling	1.5	Hr	500	750
3	Seed rate	30	Kg	120	3600
4	Sowing	1	Mandays	150	150
5	FertiliserUrea DAPMOP	70108-	KgKg	5.3624	3752592
6	Harvesting and threshing (4 cuts)	80	Man days	150	12000
7	Miscellaneous	-			-
8	Total				20717

Activities

Work out the Cost of cultivation of different kharif and rabi fodder crops.

Question

1. Why it is important to calculate the cost of cultivation of different fodder crops?

Signature of Teacher

❑❑❑

15

Livestock Waste Utilisation and Recycling

Date:

Objectives

- To get acquainted with livestock waste and about there recycling.
- To know the alternative strategies in the form of utilization of animal wastes in food production.

Material Required

- Pencil and eraser
- Models/diagrams/photographs of sheds
- Note book
- Scale.

Waste utilization and recycling

Livestock waste is of two types liquid waste (includes urine, runoff water, rain water and washing water and solid waste (includes faeces and beddings of animals).Recycling of livestock waste is very important and by recycling this waste is utilised in following practices:

- It can be applied in crop land and used as a fertilizer and thussaves money and energy otherwise spent for commercial fertilizer.
- It can be use as feed of animals (use of broiler litter in cattle feeding is a widely applied practice).
- Fuel particularly is expensive for poor households.It can be used for energy and biogas production. Thusit is used for cooking and electricity production.
- Further composting the waste also reduces the volume of the waste, hence solving serious environmental problems concerning

disposal of large quantities of waste, kills pathogens that may be present, decreases the germination of weeds in agricultural fields, and reduces offensive odour. The compost can be sold for additional revenue or used on the same farm.

Farm Yard Manure

It is a decomposed mixture of dung and urine of farm animals along with litter and left over material from roughages or fodder fed to the cattle. It is one of the components of INM it is a cheap and easily available source of organic nutrients. This source of organic improves physical, chemical and biological condition of the soils. It can supply all the nutrients required by the plant, however with low quantity.

Methods of preparation of FYM

Pit Method

This method is adopted commercially by the farmers by making usually pits of 8m x 2m x 1m dimensions these pits are filled in layers by the mixture of dung, urine and litter up to 50 cm above ground level. The top is filled and covered by dry soil and then plastered by mud paste. One pit is needed for two adult animals, the manure became ready about 150 to 180 days of plastering. One pit produced 10-12 tones of FYM or every animal gives about 5 to 6 tones of FYM / year.

Trench Method

This method is also called as Dr. C. N. Acharya method. In this method trenches of 6 to 8 m length, 1.5 to 2 m width, and 1 to 1.25 m depth are prepared. Mixture of dung and urine soaked litter is deposited in layers in these trenches until it becomes 50 cm above the ground layer. Then it is covered with 50 cm deep soil or wood ash-soil layer and then it is plastered by mud paste. Manure becomes ready for use about 150–160 days of plastering.

Heap Method

Most commonly used by the farmers. Every day sweepings, cow dung and litter are collected and heaped at one place. After about 6 to 9 months, the rotten manure is used. According to an estimate, about 30 to 35% N2, 20 to 25% P_2O_5 & 4-6% potassium are lost during preparation of manure due to leaching, washing and volatilization and other losses.

Vermicompost

Vermicomposting is a method of preparing enriched compost with the use of earthworms. It is one of the easiest methods to recycle agricultural wastes and to produce quality compost. It also called brown gold.

Vermi-composting materials are decomposable organic wastes such as animal excreta, crop residues, kitchen waste, farm residues and forest litter etc. Mixture of leguminous and non-leguminous crop residues enriches the quality of vermicompost. Different earthworms species used in vermi-composting are viz. Eisenia foetida (Red earthworm), Eudrilus eugeniae (night crawler), Perionyx excavatus etc. Among all Eisenia foetida is preferred due to its high multiplication rate and it converts the organic matter into vermicompost within 45-50 days. Since it is a surface feeder it converts organic materials into vermicompost from top.

Steps in vermicomposting

- Cattle dung is collected from cow shelters.
- The dung is kept for 7-10 days for cooling.
- Beds of dung and crop residues etc. are made about 1 m wide, 75 cm high and with a distance of 75 cm between two rows.
- In the beds, crop waste such as leaves, straw etc. is layered alternatively with the dung to thus make a height of about 75cm.
- Water is sprinkled to let the compostable matter cool down whenever desired.
- Earthworms are put on the top of the manure row. About 1 kg worms in a metre-long manure row are inoculated.
- It is left undisturbed for 2-3 days after covering with banana leaves.
- The bed is opened after 2-3 days. The upper portion of about 10 cm of manure is loosened with the help of a suitable hand tool. It also enhance aeration.

- The bed is covered again. The worms feed on an upper bed of about 10 cm. This portion becomes vermicasted in about 7-10 days.
- This portion (vermicasted manure) is removed and collected near the bed. Another upper portion of 10 cm is loosened and covered again with the leaves.
- Moisture is maintained in the bed by regular sprinkling of water.
- The loosened portion of the manure is vermicasted in another 7-10 days and is removed again.
- Thus, in about 40 days, about 60 cm of the bed is converted into vermicompost and is collected on 3-4 occasions.
- The remaining bed of about 10 cm in height contains earthworm mixed manure.
- Fresh manure mixture/organic residues, etc. are again put on the residual bed containing earthworms of about 10 cm and the composting process is restarted.
- The manure collected from the bed is freed of worms through sieving. Manual seiver or electric seiver can be used.
- The screened manure is bagged and used or sold as required.

Vermiwash

It a liquid bio-fertilizer can be collected through thecolumn of activated earthworm.It contains plant growth hormones like auxins and cytokinin apart from nitrogen, phosphorus, potash and other micronutrients. Vermiwash acts as a plant tonic and helps to reduce many plant diseases. A mixture of vermiwash (1 litre) with cow urine (1 litre) in 10 liters of water acts as biopesticide and liquid manure.

Method of vermiwash preparation

- Select large container made of concrete or plastic bucket.
- Drill a hole at the base of the container to fix a tap to it.
- Upto a base layer of gravel or broken small pieces of bricks are placed height of 10-15 cm.

- On the coarse sand layer place 40-45 cm pre-decomposed organic wastes and moisten the different layers by using water.
- Put 2000 earthworms into the container of species Eudrillus euginae or coseinea foetidae.
- The hole situated at the bottom of the pot is fixed with a water tap through whichvermiwash is collected.

Every day, the kitchen or other organic waste is put into the container. Occasionally, two or three tablespoons of fresh cowdung slurry is poured on the humus as feed for the worms. After the formation of compost, soak the entire mask with two litres of water. After 24 hours, about 1.5 litre of vermiwash can be collected.

Concentrated manures

Blood-meal when dried and powdered can be used as manure. The meat of dead animals is dried and converted into meat-meal which is a good source of nitrogen.

Nutrient content of animal based organic manures

Organic manures	Nutrient content (%)		
	N	P_2O_5	K_2O
FYM	0.5-1.5	0.4-0.8	0.5-1.9
Vermicompost	1.5	0.9	0.26
Blood meal	10-12	1-2	1.0
Meat meal	10.5	2.5	0.5
Fish meal	4-10	3-9	0.3-1.5
Horn and Hoof meal	13	-	-
Raw bone meal	3-4	20-25	-
Steamed bone meal	1-2	25-30	-

Micro-nutrient culture

Panchakavaya

It is biological plant growth promoters. It consists of five products from the cow i.e dung, urine, milk, curd and ghee. It can be kept for six months to use by stirring it daily. Recommended dose for it is 300 ml. Panchkavya liquid in 10 litreof water for all plant types.

Mudgagot

It is a natural bio-pesticide.it is a compound of cow dung, cow urine and palm sugar. After proper mixing of compounds the mud pot is closed and kept under the ground level. It can control all kind of pests in field crops. Recommended dose is 1 litre of mudgagot with 50 litres of water for all plants.

Observations

1. Visit to the vermicompost unit.

Question

1. How to make a compostwithout using earth worms?

Signature of Teacher

❑❑❑

16

Storage of Feed

Date:

Objectives

- To get acquainted with various types of storage system for minimizing the wastage coming out from feed stuffs.
- Toknow how to purchase and procure the feed.

Material Required

- Pencil and eraser
- Models/diagrams/photographs/specimens of different materials like
- Note book
- Scale.

Feeds include straw, hay, silage, grain, pellets, food by-products and un-saleable food products such asbread, fruit and vegetables, bakery productsetc. storage is very important for these feed stuffs as losses arisedue to physical and chemical changes that takes place due to improper handling also from the foraging activities of insects, micro-organisms and animals.

Following aresome of the practicesthat should be followed to control storage losses :

- Keep the storage area clean.
- Always handle feeds in a way that ensures that contamination does not occur.
- Keep the moisture level of stored feed to minimum i.e for grains less than 12% and for pulses it should be less than 10%.
- Heavily infested ingredients should not be brought into the store.
- Infested material, if accepted, should be kept separate until fumigated (this is to be done as soon as possible) to totally eradicate the pests.

- The degree of infestation can, however, is brought to manageable proportions through a programme of vigilance and effective control measures.
- Silos for grains should, therefore, be equipped with temperature sensors to provide early warning of fungal activity in stored feed-grains.
- Large stacks are advocated in the tropics to minimize weight losses.

Storage Facilities

Theseare intended to prevent losses due to leakages, rodents, and livestock, snow, rainfall, heating, insects & moulds and thusprovide easy access with regards to handling or inspecting of grain. The best storage facilities are those that are weather proof, ventilated and of single wall construction. Because small bulks cool faster and more evenly than large bulks, it is better to have several smaller bins than a few larger, ones, especially when aeration equipment is not available.

Storage structures may be made of metal or wood and regardless of the nature, they all have advantages and disadvantages. They should be built on high, well drained land in order to protect grain from heavy rainfall and spring floods. Occasionally when the crop yields are above average, grain is stored in temporary storage including barns, machine sheds or in an open area. No matter what type of structure is used to store grain, the filling should be done in the centre as this will provide even loading of the walls and a smooth uniform cone to help shed rain. Fill the granary only to the top plate to provide crawl spaces for inspection, and for ventilation. Never store newly harvested grain on top of old grain that may be infested with insects or contain spoiled grain.

Procedure

Discuss various cleaning, disinfection, storage and procurement-techniques with course instructor.

Activity

Observe and record different types of feed storage structure commonly used in Jammu region.

Questions

Whyprocurement of feed is important?

APPENDIX-1

Terminology

A.I.V method of silage making: Addition of mineral acids like sulphuric acid and hydrochloric acid is used to bring the pH below 4.0.

Fertilizer : It is an organic or inorganic substance added to soil to increase the plant growth.

Fertiliser analysis: It expresses weight as a percent of N,P and K.

Fertilizer Use Efficiency: It is extent of fertilizer use recovery in agriculture per crop unit.

Fodder crops are those crops which are cultivated primarily for animal feed.

Forage is a plant material (mainly plant leaves and stems) eaten by grazing livestock·Historically, the term forage has meant only plants eaten by the animals directly as pasture, crop residue, or immature cereal crops, but it is also used more loosely to include similar plants cut for fodder and carried to the animals, especially as hay.

Hay: it is a stored forage that has been cut and dried with 10-15 % moisture content.

Haylage: It is grown and cut similar to hay but it is baled before it is dry, mostly when there is 35-40% moisture content.

Pasture and range land Includes all forage feeds either not cut (including feeds cured on the stem) or cut and fed fresh (greenchop or silage).

Silage: it is fermented high moisture (75%) stored fodder.

Silpauline is a polythene tarpaulin which is resistant to the ultra violet radiation in sunlight.

Wastelage: Waste material (animal organic waste) in suitable combinations with forage and additive, under anaerobic conditions, through fermentation by lactic acid producing bacteria.

Appendix-2

Type	Name of crop	Botanical name
Grasses		
	Senji	*Malilotus parviflora*
	Buffal grass	*Cenchrus ciliaris*
	Jerga grass	*Dicanthium annulatum*
	Rhodes grass	*Chloris gayana*
	Blue panic	*Panicum antidotale*
	Dub grass	*Cynodon dactylon*
	Para grass	*Brachiara mutica*
	Kikuya grass	*Pennisetum clandestinum*
	Sewan	*Lasiurus sindicus*
Leguminous fodder		
	Tall Fescue	*Festuca arundinacea*
	Perennial rye grass	*Lolium perennea*
	Moth	*Phaseolusaconitifolius*
	Stylo	*Stylosanthes gracilis*
	Cocks foot	*Doctylus glomierata*
	Dallis grass	*Paspalum dilatatum*
	Kala Dhaman	*Cenchrus setigerus*

Appendix-3

Agronomical practices for production of fodders

Kharif cereals

Practices	Sorghum (Jowar,Chari)	Maize (Makka)	Teosinite (Makchari)	Bajra (Pearl millet)	Pioneer Jowar
Botanical name	*Sorghum bicolour*	*Zea mays*	*Zea mexicana*	*Pennisetumglaucum*	
Crop varieties	Ujjain,swarna-413,M.P. charri,PC - 6,PC-23,S-194,Hara sona, HC-136	African tall, Vijay, Kissan, Ganga, HGT-3, Jawahar, Ganga 2,3,5	Sirsa improved	S530,Giant,Rajko,K5 99,T-55,Ap. Complex, L-72, L-74, K-674	Hybrid variety
Sowing time	April-May(sub-temperate) July (sub-tropical)	June-August	March-August	April-May and extend to mid July	March-July(irrigated) July (un-irrigated)
Seed rate(kg/ha)	50-60	50-60	40-50	10	25-30
Method	Broad casted	Broad casted	Broad casted	Broad casted	Broad casted
Manures and fertilizers FYM(t/ha) N (kg/ha) P(kg/ha) K(kg/ha)	(single cut) (multi cut) 7-10 210 90 60 30 60	 60-120 40-60 40	40 50 40-50 30-40	7-10 60 40	60 kg urea,125 kg DAP as basal ,each cut is followed by 75 kg urea/ha
Irrigation interval (days)	10-15	7-10	15-20	15-20	-
Period of harvesting(days)	After 80 days, 50-55 days (M.P. charri) (subsequent 35-40 days)	70-75	60-70 (subsequent 80-90 days) 7-10 days before	60 (subsequent 35-40 days) Harvested at boot or 50% below early	40(subsequent 25-30 days)
No. of cuttings	2-3 (multi cut)	1	2	2	2-3
Yield(q/ha)	300-350	400-500	400-500	400-500	400-500
Miscella-neous	HCN (during) Poisioning		x2 tasseling		

Khariflegumes

Practices	**Lucern** (Alfalfa)	**Cowpea (**Lobia)	**Clusterbean (Guara)**
Botanical name	*Medicago sativa*	*Vigna unguiculata*	*Cyamopsis tetragonaloba*
Crop varieties	Sirsa-8, sirsa-9 T-9	EC 4216, HF-642-1, TYPE 2 K-395	FS-277, Ageta Guara-III Guaea-80
Sowing time	April-May (temperate) July-August (Summer) September-November (Autumn)	April-July	June-August
Seed rate(kg/ha)	15-20	50-60	40-50
Method	Broadcasting	Broadcasting	Broadcasting
Manures and fertilizers			
FYM	5-6 t/ha		
N	5	40	10-15
P	60	60	20-25
K			
Irrigation interval(days)	10-15	2-3 irrigations are required	No irrigation after 3rd week of September
Period of harvesting(days)	70-90(subsequent 30-45 days)	60-70	Pods begin
No. of cuttings	6-7		Till the pods are fully formed
Yield(q/ha)	600-800/year	150-200	300-450

Kharif (Grasses)

Practices	Deenanath	Setaria grass	Hybrid napier
Crop varieties	PP15, IGFRI-43-1, PP-10, PS-3, IGFRI-4-22-1, S-56-1, Bundel-1	Nandi, Kazungula Narok, Splenda	Pusa , Giant, N.B.21, IGFRI-10, BN-2, Co-1, IGFRI-6, CO-2, CO-3, APBN-1
Sowing time	April –May (irrigated) Monsoon (rain fed)	February	February-MarchMid June- end July
Seed rate	7.5 kg/ha	33,500-67000 root slips	18,000-20,000
Method	Broadcasting	50X30 cm spacing	60X80 cm
Manures and fertilizers			
FYM	200q	125-200q	
N	60	60	250
P	40	40	50
K	15	40	50
Irrigation interval(days)	10	7-10 days	10-15
Period of harvesting(days)	100	80(subsequent 6-8 weeks)	50-60(subsequent 30-35 days)
No. of cuttings	>3	>7	5-6
Yield	300q/ha for 3 cuts	900q/ha for 7 cuts	1000-1150q/ ha/year

Rabi fodder

Practices	Cereals	Legumes	Brassica
Fodder	**Oats (Jai)**	**Berseem (Egyptian clover)**	**Sarson (Chinese cabbage)**
Botanical name	*Avena sativa*	*Trifolium alexandrinum*	*Brassica pekinensis*
Crop varieties	Kent, Sabzar, Black nip, HFD-114	Mescavi, vardhan, BL-1, 2, 10, 22, 42	Chinese cabbage F-2-902, 916
Sowing time	October-November	September-October	1st fortnight of October
Seed rate(Kg/ha)	100	25-30	6-7
Method	Line sowing (20-25 cm apart)	Broadcasting	25 cm apart
Manures and fertilizers			
FYM(t/ha)	15-20t	25	40
N(kg/ha)	90-120	50	20
P(kg/ha)	30-40	50	10
K(kg/ha)	20		
Irrigation interval (days)	15-20	8-10(winter) 6-7(summer)	15-20
Period of harvesting(days)	60-75 (subseq-uent 40-50)	45(subseq-uent 25-40)	50-60
No. of cuttings	2	4-5	1
Yield(q/ha)	400-500	700-800	200-300
Miscellaneous		Cause blotting	

Signature of Teacher

❑❑❑

17

General Managment Practices in Farm Animals

Date:

Objective

To get acquainted with general management practices like disbudding, washing, grooming, exercise, dipping, spraying, clipping, shearing, training of breeding bulls etc.

Material Recquired

Disbudding equipment, brushes, bull exerciser, dipping tub/tank sprayer, scissor, shearers, rope and other restraining equipments.

Procedure

1. DISBUDDING

Disbudding which is a pre-requisite of a loose housing system to prevent fight, damage to structures/attendants can be done between 7-10 days in buffalo calves and 10-15 days in cow calves or later with the help of hot iron dis-budder or electric dis-budder or caustic stick.

In case of hot iron dis-budder:

1. Remove the hair at the point of bud
2. Restrain the calf properly
3. Burn the bud with hot iron dis-budder till the bud is completely burnt
4. Apply antiseptic cream tills the wound heals up.

2. WASHING

In general washing/cleaning of animals is required for clean milk production, to get rid heat stress in summers. Buffalo is a water loving animal. This can be done once/twice per day depending upon the requirement.

3. GROOMING

It can be done with the help of brushes like soft dandy brushes comparatively hard nylon brush and curry comb to stimulate blood circulation, removal of ecto-parasites and removal of dust, dirt and dung etc. It can be done at least once a day.

4. EXERCISE

It is an important aspect in breeding bulls for increased quantity as well as quality of semen. They require at least one hour exercise daily which should be provided in cool hours. This can be done with the help of bull exercisers.

5. DIPPING

It is a technique to immerse the animal completely in the dip containing insecticides/pesticides for killing ecto parasites, particularly in sheep.

Generally done once/twice per year but frequency may be more depending upon infestation.

6. SPRAYING

If the flock is small, then instead of dipping spraying with the help of spray pump is preferred to economize resources.

7. CLIPPING

Removal/thinning of hairs from body coat with the help of clippers in many domesticated animals before the start of summer or at the end of rainy season is done to lessen the heat load and for the growth of fresh hair.

8. SHEARING

It is removal of wool fibre from the body of sheep which is primarily done for economic reasons. Besides it decreases heat stress, kills ecto-parasites and temporarily more number of animals can be accommodated in same space. It can be done once/twice in a year with the help of traditional shear or electric shearing.

9. TRAINING OF BREEDING BULLS

Generally it is done from the age of two years & onward. It is a particularly important for bulls used for semen collection with regard to mounting on dummy and ejaculating in artificial vagina.

Assignment

Observe and practice different management practices without disturbing the regular schedule of the live stock farm.

Questions

1. Why disbudding with hot iron dis-budder is preferred as compared to other methods?
2. What will be the effect if proper exercise and training is not given to breeding bulls?

Signature of Teacher

❑❑❑

18

Milking of Dairy Animals

Date:

Objectives

1. To get familiarize with different milking techniques.
2. To observe the various management practices adopted for higher and clean milk production.

Material Required

Visit to different types of milking parlors, photographs, diagrams showing different types of milking techniques.

Prerequisite

Knowledge or information on following aspects is required

a) Application of milk man's knot - For restraining the animal

b) Type of dairy cattle housing - Conventional-loose/semi loose

c) Type of milking parlor
- Abreast
- Tandem
- Herring bone
- Rotary

d) Milking technique
- Full hand milking
- Stripping
- Machine milking

e) Mechanism of milk secretion

Procedure

HAND MILKING

1. In general the animals should be washed and cleaned while shifting them from their shed to milking parlor. This will depend upon season and cleanliness of animal.
2. Feed the animal with required quantity of concentrate.
3. Wash the udder with clean water and dry it with a piece of clean cloth. $KMnO_4$ can also be added in water.
4. The milker should wash and dry his hand thoroughly before milking.
5. Prepare the animal for milk let down by manipulating the udder, teats and with other routine practices.
6. Milk the animal with full palm method.
7. Strain the milk after complete milking.
8. Keep the milk in a cool place.

Machine Milking

1. Preliminary step up to washing of udder will remain same.
2. Observe and practice the application of cups on teats
3. Remove the cups at the end of milking.
4. Release the animals from the milking parlour.

Stripping Method

The last strips of milking, in case of hand milking as well as in some kind of machine milking and in those cases where teats are very small milk is removed with the help of thumb along with fore finger and middle finger.

Precautions

- Do not make any noise in the milking parlor
- Do not beat or disturb the animals at the time of milking.
- Do not feed the silage or duty feed at milking time.

Assignments

1. Record milk let down time, type and quantity of feed offered, quantity of milk produced of at least 2 animals.
2. Practice hand milking.

Questions

1. What do you mean by withholding-up of milk?
2. What is pulsation rate and pulsation ratio?
3. What is the difference in the principle for hand milking and machine milkilng?

Signature of Teacher

❑❑❑

19

Layout Plans for Housing of Cattle and Buffalo

Date:

Objective

a) To effectively use available land resources
b) To provide proper animal comfort, ventilation and sanitation
c) Proper planning for improvement of farm productivity
d) Better management of livestock
e) It helps for construction of cost effective houses
f) Future expansion of the farm.

Housing Plan for Livestock

Selection of site for farm building

Proper housing which is conducive to good health, comfort and protection from inclement weather and which would enable the animals to utilize their genetic ability and feed for optimal production. Before selecting a site the following points are to be considered.

Soil

Soil must be suitable for strong foundation. Marchy, clay, sandy, rock soils are not suitable. Loamy and gravely soils are best suited for building construction.

Availability of land

There should be vast area to construct all building and should give way to future expansion of farm. Atleast 2-3 acre land is required for 200 cows accommodation. For 2 cows 1acre land is essential for fodder production.

Drainage system

Proper drainage of rain and subsoil water should be provided to keep healthy environment and to protect the building from dampness.

Availability of water

Plenty of water is needed for farm operations like washing, fodder cultivation, processing of milk and byproducts and for drinking.

Sun Shade

With the east-west orientation the feed and water troughs can be under the shade .The shaded area, however, should be increased to 3 to 4m^2 per cow. By locating the feed and water in the shade, feed consumption will be encouraged, but also more manure will be dropped in the shaded area which in turn will lead to dirty cows.

With the north-south orientation, the sun will strike every part of the floor area under and on either side of the roof at some time during the day. This will help to keep the floored area dry. A shaded area of 2.5 to 3m^2 per cow is adequate if feed and water troughs are placed away from the shaded area.

In regions where temperatures average 30°C or more for up to five hours per day during some period of the year, the east-west orientation is most beneficial.

Electricity

It is needed for operating various machines used in the farm and is the light source to the animals and should be available.

Protection from wind and solar radiation

If the farm building in open or exposed area, the wind breaks in the farm of tall quick growing trees should be grown near the building.

Protection from noise and other disturbance

The farm site should be away from noise producing factory/ chemical industry, sewage disposing area. The industrial effluents in the form of gaseous or liquid may pollute surrounding resources.

Availability of market facility

The farm should be away from the city but at the same time it should be nearer to city thereby the products produced from the farm could be marketed easily.

Transport facility

The farm buildings should be provided with good road and also have the accessibility to reach the market to reduce the transport cost and avoid spoilage of products.

Layout of Dairy Farm

It includes the following

1. Location and grouping of farm buildings.
2. Location of pathways and roads.
3. Division of farm land into plots.

Distribution of land of dairy farm

a)	Land under Buildings, Paddocks and roads	: 8%
b)	Land under fodder cultivation	: 80%
c)	Land under permanent pasture	: 8%
d)	Land under cash crops	: 4%

a) **Pathways and roads:**

Pathways must connect each building of cattle yard, offices, residential quarters etc. Roads must be well graveled for quick transport. As far as possible, roads must be straight for easy and economic haulage. Layout of roads must be such which requires minimum wastage of land.

b) **Fodder fields and Pastures:**

Number and size of plots must be according to cropping rotations/plan. All plots must be well connected to roads and irrigation channels. Layout of plots must be such that it is easy to irrigate without soil erosion.

c) **Dairy farm building:**

Dairy cow building must have following parts

- Feeding passage
- Manger
- Standing space
- Gutter or drainage channel
- Milking passage

Main building units

- Milking barn or parlour
- Down calver shed/calving pen
- Calf pen
- Young stock or heifer shed
- Dry animal shed
- Bull shed
- Isolation shed
- Quarantine shed
- Store room
- Milk room
- Hay or straw shed

The layout of dairy farm buildings for 200 cows and followers is presented below:

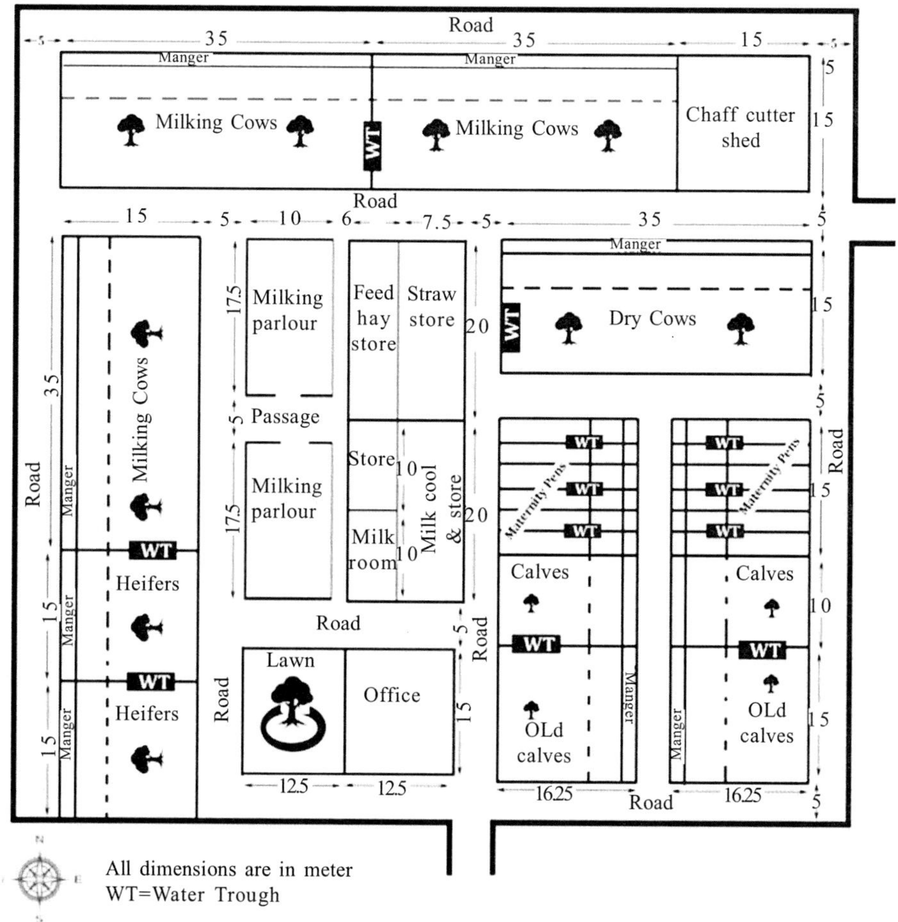

Floor space requirements

Type of animal	Floor space requirement (m²)		Max. no of animals / pen	Height of the shed (cm)
	Covered area	Open area		
Bulls	12.0	24.0	1	175 cm. in medium and heavy rain fall and 220 cm. in dry areas.
Cows	3.5	7.0	50	
Buffaloes	4.0	8.0	50	
Down – calver	12.0	12.0	1	
Young – calves	1.0	2.0	30	
Old – calves	2.0	4.0	30	

Feeding and watering space requirements

Type of animal	Space per animal (cm)	Manger length/ 100 animals(cm)	Water tank length for 100 animals (cm)
Adult cattle & buffaloes	60 – 75	6000 – 7500	600 – 750
Calves	40 – 50	4000 – 5000	400 – 500

Dimensions of feed manger

Type of animal	Width (cm)	Depth (cm)	Height of inner wall (cm)
Adult cattle and buffaloes	60	40	50
Calves	40	15	20

Main Building Units

1. Dairy cow building

The milch animal shed should have the following parts

- Feeding passage
- Manger
- Standing space
- Gutter or drainage channel
- Milking passage

The animals can be kept in single row system if numbers of animals are small (12-16 no.) or in double row system (16-50 nos.). The distance between two sheds should be greater than 30 feet or it should be twice the height of the building.

In double row system two methods available

1. **Tail to tail system:** In this system animals in two rows faces opposite to each other. Main advantages of this system are easy cleaning and milking of animals, less chance for transmission of diseases from animal to animal, and animals can get more fresh air from outside.

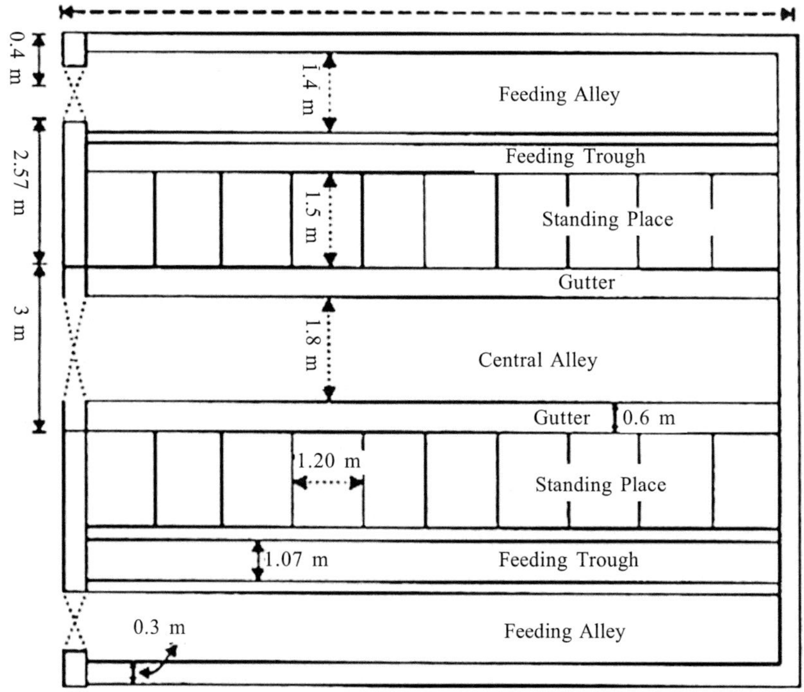

Top view of Tail-to- tail system of housing

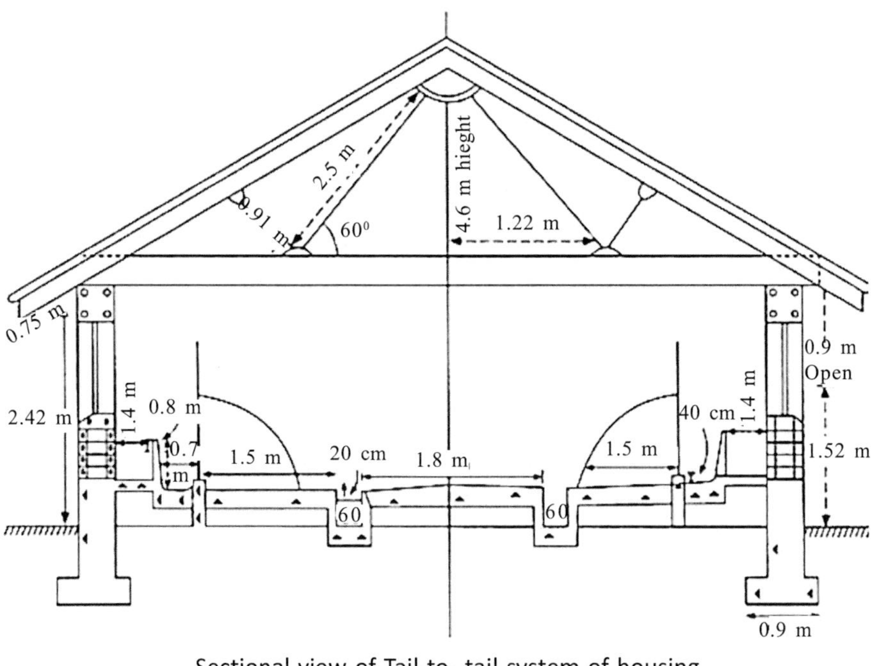

Sectional view of Tail-to- tail system of housing
Graphics Compiled and edited from Web Resource

2. **Head to head system:** In this system animals in two rows faces each other. Main advantages of this system are getting animals into the shed is easy.Feeding of animals also easy.Disinfection of gutter will be more due to the direct fall of sunrays over the gutter.Animals are better exhibited to visitors. However, milking supervision is difficult in this system and possibilities of transmission of disease are more.

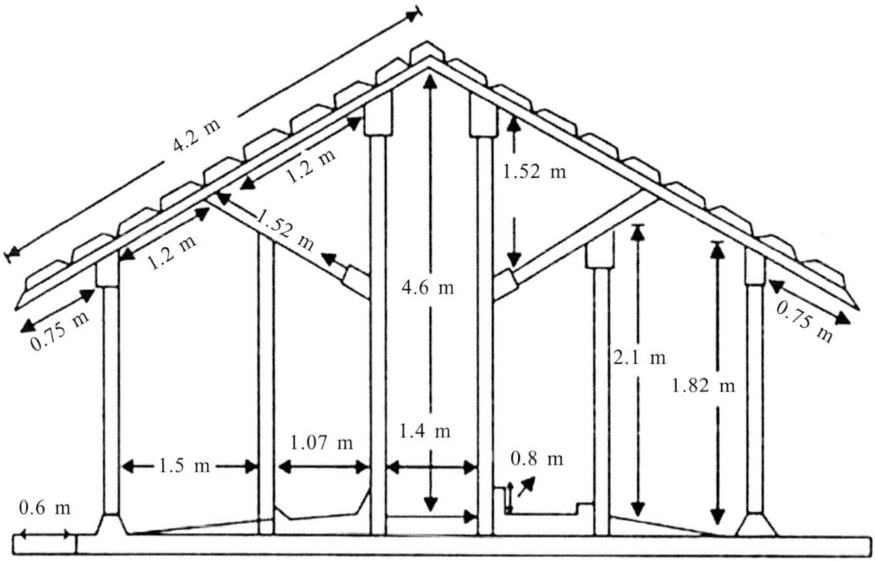

Sectional view of head-to- head system of housing
Graphics Compiled and edited from Web Resource

a) Milking barn or parlour

This is a fully covered barn where milch animals are milked.It should be located at the centre of the farm with all other farm buildings arranged around it.There shall be an individual standing in the milking barns and the number of standings required should be 25% of total number of milch animals in the herd.

Dimensions of milking barn

- Standing space : 1.5 - 1.7 m (L) × 1.05 - 1.2m (W)
- Width of central passage : 1.5 - 1.8 m
- Width of feed alley : 0.75 m
- Width of gutter : 0.30 m
- Overhang : 0.75 m

b) Down calver shed/ calving pen

Pregnant animals are transferred to a calving pen 2 to 3 weeks before the expected date of calving. Calving pen of 3m x 4m (12 m^2) is essential to keep the animals in advanced stage of pregnancy. It should be located nearer to the farmer's quarters for better supervision.The number of calving pens required is 10% of the number of total breedable female stock in the farm.

c) Calf pen

This is meant for housing young calves separately. If calves are not weaned immediately after birth and are allowed for suckling, it can be located either at the end or on the side of the milking barn. This facilitates taking calves to their dams quickly.

If calves are weaned at birth and there are large numbers of calves, the separate unit of calf shed should be arranged and could be located nearer to the maternity pens.

Recommended floor space requirement for different age group of calves

Age of Calves (months)	Floor space requirement covered area (m_2)	Floor space requirement open area (m_2)	Number of calvesper pen
0-3	1.0	2	30
3-6	1.5	3	30
6-12	2.0	4	12

d) Young stock/ heifer shed

It is meant for housing young heifers separately.Older heifers calves from about six months of age to breeding age are to be housed separately from the suckling calves.When a large number of young stocks are there, they should be divided into different age groups and each group housed separately.

e) Dry animal shed

Normally, one third of the animals in a farm will be in dry or in dry cum pregnant stage. In large farms, milch and dry cows are housed separately. The floor in the covered area should preferably be made of cement concrete. Under Indian conditions, in smaller farms, milch and dry animals can be housed together.

f) Bull shed

Floor space requirement: In the covered area 12m^2 per bull can be provided and the open exercise yard 120m^2 per bull. If open yard is not provided the bull exerciser is needed.

Wall: The solid wall should be constructed with the height of 1.5 meter and above these walls two or three horizontal tubular rods with the gap of 20 to 30 cm are fixed.

Floor: Floor can be constructed with rough cement concrete and should have a gradient slope of 1/40 to 1/60 to have easy accessibility to the drainage channel.

Roof: Gable or monitor roof with eaves of 2.5 - 3 m height should be provided and ridge height should be 3.2 - 3.5 m.

Manger: A cement concrete manger with the dimension of 60 cm width, 40 cm depth and 50 cm height of inner wall should be provided inside the bull shed. The bull shed should have a water trough with the dimension of about 60 to 75 cm length.

Yard: A yard is an open area for the bull and should be of 120m^2 and the yard should be enclosed on all sides by 0.3 m solid wall and iron tubular rods as partitions to a height of 1.2 m placed at 0.25 m intervals.

g) Isolation shed

It is the separation of sick animals from apparently healthy animals to avoid transmission of diseases to healthy stock.It should be located at the corner of the shed.

Accessory buildings

a) **Store room:** All the four walls should be closed and it should be rat proof. There should be one concrete store room with feed mixing unit at a distant place and a smaller feed store room behind the milking parlour.

b) **Milk room:** It is essential to keep the milk and also to chill the milk in larger dairies having 400 to 700 litres production capacity that requires 3.7 m x 5m size of room and an additional 0.37 m^2 for every 40 litres of milk production. For a smaller dairy unit below 100 litres a small room with a dimension of 3.75m x 3m can be sufficient for storing milk and concentrate feed.

c) **Hay or straw shed:** An adult animal consume about 5 to 10 kg of hay or straw per day, while young stock consume about 2 to 5 kg of hay or straw per day. The annual requirement can be calculated and the space requirement can be arrived.

Assignments

Prepare a layout plan for housing of 100 cows and followers. Sketch the top and sectional view of main dairy building in tail to tail system with dimensions.

Questions

1. Draw the manger (adult animals) as per given specifications.
2. Provide the space requirements of different category of dairy animals.
3. Discuss the merits and demerits of tail to tail system of housing.

Signature of Teacher

❑❑❑

20

Layout Plans for Housing of Sheep and Goat

Date:

Objective

1. To provide shelter from heat, cold, rain and draught
2. Provide comfort to the animals
3. Increase efficiency in management of animals
4. Protection from wild animals.

Selection of site for farm building

S.No	Factors	Desired characteristics	Required for
1.	Site	i. Easily approachable	To supervise and take care
		ii. Spacious	For future expansion
2.	Soil	i. Sandy loam	For proper drainage to keep the surrounding clean and dry
		ii. fertile	For good yield of fodder
		iii. Condition- neither too dry nor too moist	For longer life of shed
3.	Topography	Elevated (high, level without abrupt slope)	i. Low cost of construction ii. Effective drainage
4.	Sunlight	Exposure of floor to sunlight	i. Keep the floor and building clean. ii. Check germ growth
5.	Winds	No direct draft of hot and cold wind Planting trees as wind breakers	i. To provide shade and cool environment ii. To prevent sudden change in temperature

6.	Market	Nearby	i. Quick disposal of farm product ii. Quick procurement of raw material iii. To minimize cost of transportation
7.	Water	Enough and continuous	i. To meet the water requirement of animals ii. To keep the farm premise clean
8.	Other factors	i. Telephone ii. Nearby school for children of farm workers iii. Post office iv. Shopping centre	For the welfare of the employees

Sheep are reared for meat or wool or both. Goat are reared for meat or milk or both. Requirement for building units are more or less same for sheep and goat. Additional buildings are required for goats kept for milk.

Building for sheep and goat

1. Shed

i) General flock shed (15m x 4m x 3m) : For housing of adult breeding ewes and nannies

ii) Shed for ram or buck (2.25m x 1.5m x 3m) : For housing of rams or bucks individually.

iii) Lambing or kidding shed (1.5m x 1.2m x 3m) : For housing of pregnant ewes or nannies are housed individually.

iv) Lamb or kid shed (7.5m x 4m x 3m) : For housing of lambs or kids from weaning upto maturity.

v) Sick animal shed (3m x 2m x 3m) : Sick animals are housed individually in this shed. It should be constructed away from the animal shed.

2. Shepherds house

It is meant for the caretaker. It should be located at a convenient place in the yard.

3. Accessory Buildings

i) Stores: (a) Storing concentrate, straw and farm equipments (b) Weighing yard

4. Requirement for sheep farm

i) Shearing room (6m x 2.5m x 3m)-Required in farms where sheep are reared for wool. This room should be well-lit by having large glass windows all around. The floor should be cement paved and surface smooth. On either side of shearing room there should be holding pens where sheep can be collected before and after shearing. These lots should lead into the shearing room through 1.5m wide passage. Next to the shearing room should be the wool store room for storing wool and equipments

ii) Dipping tank

5. Buildings for milch goat farm

I. Shed

- i) Milch goat shed: The milch goat shed should be divided into a number of stalls, one stall for each doe. This facilitates milking and stall feeding of goats individually.
- ii) Buck shed
- iii) Kidding shed
- iv) Kid shed

II. Milking room

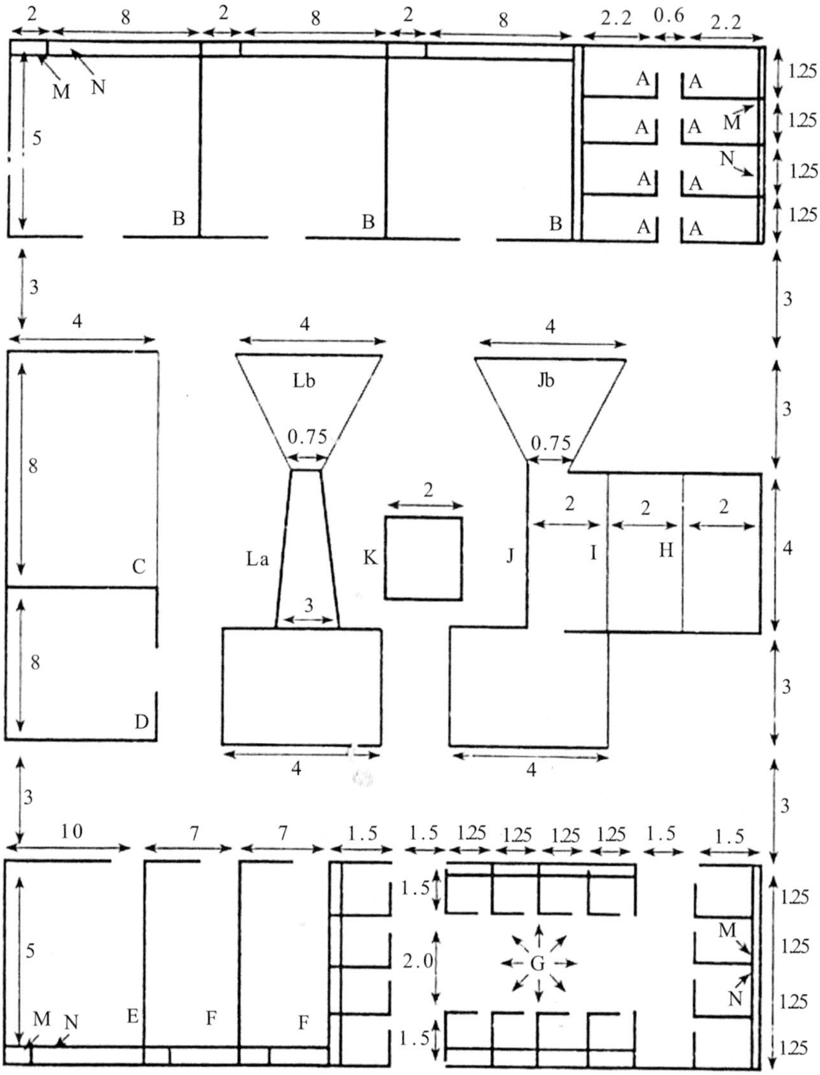

A. Ram/Buck pens, B. Ewe (Nanny) pens, C. Hay/straw shed, D. Store, E. Older (or market) lamb/kid pen, F. Weaner lambs, kid shed, G. Lambing/kidding-Cum-sick animal pen, H. Office. I. Wool store, Ja.Shearing room Jb. Assembly pen. Jc. Collecting pen, K. Dipping gear store, La. Dipping tank, Lb. Holding pen, Lc. Draining pen M. Water tank (1/10th length of manger in each pen), N. Manger. (In case of milch goat farms the milk doe stalls can be raised in place of the shearing room).

Layout plan for housing 200 ewes/does

Graphic Source : Web Resource

Construction details of the Units

The shed should be constructed in E-W orientation for providing cooler environment within the shed. The house should be semi close type *i.e.* E-W there should be complete wall upto roof and towards N-S it should be semi closed type *i.e* wall upto half of its height. The most appropriate height is 3m in the centre and 2m on the sides. There must be an open space in front of each animal shed. Open space requirement per animal is double to that of covered space.

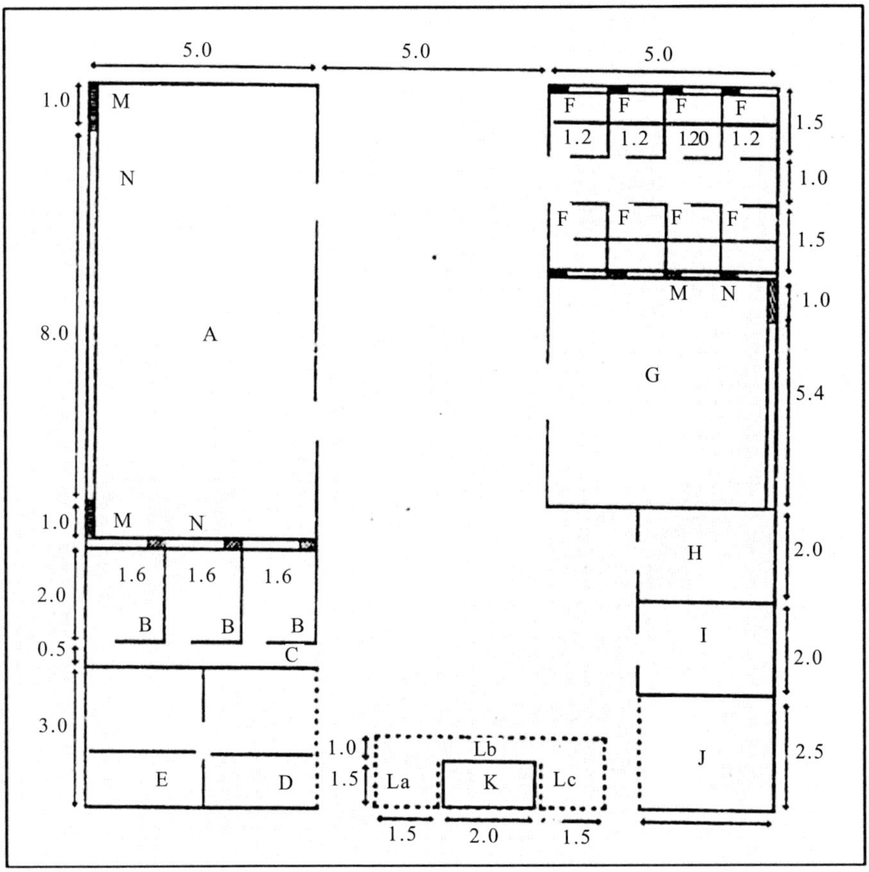

A. Ewe (Nanny) pens, B. Ram/Buck pens, C. Passage leading to ram/buck pens, D. Shearing room, E. Wool store, F. Lambing/kidding pens, G. Lamb/kid pen, H. Office, I. Store, J. Hay/straw shed, K. Hand dipping tank (1m deep), La. Assembly pen, Lb. Corridor for sheep movement, Lc. Draining pen, M. Water tank (1/10th length of manger in each pen), N. Manager. (In case of milch goat farms, the milk doe stalls can be raised in place of the shearing room).

Layout plan for housing 50 ewes/does

Graphic Source : Web Resource

1. Floor : It may be either of moorum or of strong wooden batten in areas of heavy rainfall. In the case of wooden batten flooring, the width of each plank shall vary from 75-100mm and the thickness between 25 and 40 mm. The sides of the plank shall be well rounded and the clearance between two plank shall range between 10 to 15 mm to facilitate the disposal of dung and urine. The wooded batten floor shall be constructed at a height of at least 1m above the ground level. In this case a suitable ramp or steps of wooden plank shall be provided. For shearing room/ store room/shepherd house flooring may be moorum/brick in cement morter and be properly levelled. The floor should be kachha or sandy under hot dry conditions of arid or semi arid areas. A suitable drain should be provided at the end of the floor. The depth of the drain should be 75 mm and width 300 to 400 mm.

2. Walls : The walls may be of brick in lime morter up to two-third of their height from the floor level. The upper one third portion of the walls may be of bird proof netting.

3. Roof : The roof may be lean-to or gabled type. The slope of the roof shall depend upon rainfall and other climatic conditions of the region. The roof may be made of plain or corrugated asbestos cement sheet, plain or corrugated galvanized steel sheet, aluminum sheet or thatch. In thatched roof the thickness shall be atleast 15 mm. The eaves of the roof shall project out sufficiently long to prevent rain water entering into the house.

4. Gate : Each shed may be provided with one or more gates either on long or broad sides of the sheds depending upon the dimension of the shed. The dimension of each gate may be 0.8m broad and 1m high. The gate leaf and frame may be made of wooden batten.

5. Manger : The manger may be either of cement concrete or of wood with two compartments for providing feed and hay. A separate hay rack may also be provided by fixing at level or slightly below the heads of the animals. The water trough may be of cement concrete or galvanised steel pails or buckets and may be fixed or hung from a hook fixed to the walls. The manger may also be of portable type. The number of mangers and water trough in each shed may vary according to the number of animals.

6. Dipping tank : The dipping tank to protect the animals from ectoparasites may be made either of galvanised steel sheets or constructed of stone or brick in cement morter. If galvanised steel tank is used, it shall be well bedded down and the soil rammed tight against it to prevent the sides of thebath from bulging when it is filled. The dipping tank may be at one side of the yard
7. Foot bath : A foot bath made of galvanised steel sheets or brick in cement morter shall be provided at the entrance to the yard to protect the animals from foot rot disease.

Housing of goats kept for milk production

The type of housing for the goats may have the following units

I. Shed

II. Milk room

III. Store room

i) Dairy goat shed : The shed shall consist of stall for keeping the milking doe. The stalls shall be arranged in two rows with a passage in between them. The dimension of each stall meant to keep a single milking doe may be 1.2m wide and1.4m long. The length of the shed shall depend upon the number of milking doe kept for milk production. There shall be partitions separating one stall from the other.

ii) Buck shed : There shall be partition of wooden planks to divide the shed into compartment for housing bucks individually. The buck shed shall be away from milk room and kidding shed.

iii) Kid shed : A shed used to accommodate young goats

iv) Kidding shed : A shed used as maternity room for doe

v) Milk room : A room where excess of milk is kept for disposal and sometimes used for milking does.

vi) Store room : For storing feed and other material.

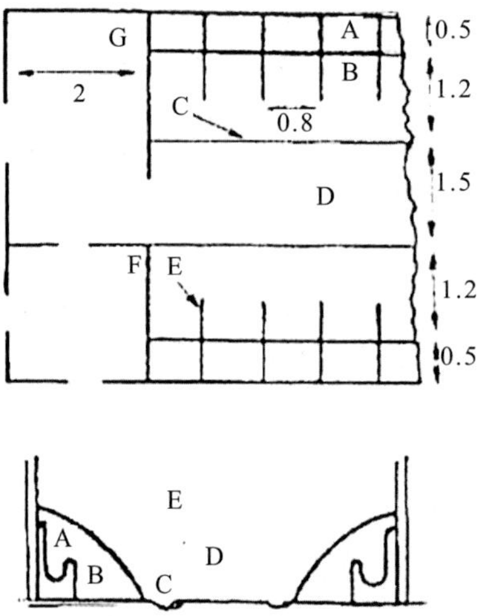

A. Manger. B. Standing space. C. Gutter, D. Central passage, E. Iron tubing partition between two stalls, F. Store, G. Milk house.

Details of stalls for milch goats

Table 1. Minimum floor space requirement per animal and maximum numbers of animals that can be housed in one shed

S.No	Type of animal	Min floor space/ animal m^2	Max animal/shed
1.	Ewe/doe	1.0	60
2	Ram/Buck	3.2	1
3	Lamb/Kid	0.4	75
4.	Weaner	0.8	75
5.	Weaner	0.9	1
6.	Ewe with lamb	1.5	1

Feeding and watering space requirement

Type of animal	Space per animal (cm)	Width of manger/ water trough(cm)	Depth of manger/ water trough (cm)	Height of inner wall of manger/water trough (cm)
Sheep and goat	40 - 50	50	30	35
Kid/lamb	30 - 35	50	20	25

Questions

1. Draw a lay-out plan of goat/sheep farm for 20 ewes/does, 1 ram/buck and 30 kids
2. Write short notes on: (a) Lean-to-type shed (b) Slatted floor house.

Signature of Teacher

❑❑❑

21

Approaching, Handling and Restraining of Cattle and Buffalo

Date:

Objective

To approach, handle and restrain an animal for different managemental practices to be carried on the animal.

Principles of approaching and handling

Remain together as a flock or herd is a social behavior of most of the domestic animals. This instinct of grouping together is very strong in sheep, less in cattle and pigs. Therefore, it is difficult to separate a sheep from the flock, but easy to separate a cow or pig. The response of animals to handling depends on their sensory capabilities Cattle, sheep, and pigs are able to hear higher frequency sounds than human do and it is possible for the animals to become fearful of sounds which we cannot even hear. Most of the human ear are sensitive at 1000-3000 Hz but cattle are most sensitive to 8000 Hz, and can easily hear upto 21000 Hz.

Another important concept in approaching animals is the flight zone of the animal when handlers approach individuals or group of animals, the animals react by observing the persons movement and then turning a way to escape. The distance at which animals react by fleeing is the "flight distance" and the area inside that distance the "flight zone" Entering the flight zone of animal from causes it to back away or turn before fleeing. The visual field of animals is also important. Cattle have wide angle (306°) panoramic vision and they can see colour. To avoid and too strong a reaction by the animal, handlers are advised to work on the edge of the flight zone, and avoid conspicuous movements.

Cattle sheep, goat, buffaloes, horses are more docile than that of pig and canine. Age sex and physiological condition will also affect the behavior of animals during handling and transport. Castrated animals are easier to handle than intact animals. Females behave differently when they are in estrous or near parturition. Animals will behave differently depending on their previous experience. Animals should not be pushed to an extreme emotion.

Material Required

Animals, bull nose ring, bull nose punch, bull holder, bull leader, muzzle, ropes of different sizes and crush.

Prerequisite

Basic knowledge regarding general behaviour of the species/ animal to be handled.

Procedure

1. **Approaching:**

   In most of the species, approach from the front side and go near the left side of the animal very cautiously and gently. Generally, milking is done from left side and identification mark is also present on left side. Never approach from rear side because the animal may get frightened and may kick, may harm with movement of tail or may hurt with the head. Therefore, get familiar with the animal by approaching from front side and then patting on its neck or shoulder.

2. **Handling and Restraining:**

   Despite the fact that some improved and modern techniques are available for handling the animal but the ropes are still used to handle and restrain the animals in the field because of economic reasons and convenience. These ropes can be of different materials like nylon, coconut, jute and cotton etc. They are with different thickness represented by strands.

Restraining of cattle & buffaloes

Temporary Restrains

Tail restraint: Both hands are kept close to the base of the tail, and the tail is trained upward without cursing any injury. The operator should stand to one side to avoid kicking by the cow.

Nose lead: It is applied at the nose of the animal and then the rope is pulled and tied to the pole, if needed.

Manual restraint of head: The nasal septum is firmly grasped with the thumb and fore-finger with one hand and horn or ear with the other.

Ear twitch: A loop is formed around the horns and the rope is carried around the ear and the end of the rope is passed under the standing part to form a half hitch. The end of the rope is then pulled to apply restraint.

Restrains for prevent kicking

Milking restraint: A rope one meter in length is tied to the hind limbs above the hock by crossing its end

Squeeze restraint: A loop is formed around the animals body infront of udder/prepuce with a rope having an eye at one end. The end of the rope is pulled tight to that the rope squeezes the animal.

Methods to raise a leg

Raising a fore limb: The leg can be raised manually provided the animal is docile and the operator is physically strong. The leg can be raised with the help of a rope having an eye at one end. A loop is formed around the pastern and the other end of the rope passed over the withers and is held by an assistant.

Raising a hind limb: The hind limb can also be raised manually. The leg is grasped at the pastern with left hand and the animals flank is pushed with the operator's shoulder so as to shift weight of the animals to the other leg (Fig 2.29). At this time leg is raised and the position of the limb is so adjusted so as to hold its weight on the operator's leg.

Casting restraint

Burely methods/Alternative method

A 12-15m long rope is doubled and its center is places over the withers of the animal. The ends of the roped are carried between the forelimbs and crossed at the sternum. One end is carried up each side of the animals body and the ends are again crossed over the back. The ends are now passed between the medical surface of the rear legs.

The ends of the rope are pulled to cast the animal. The tail is pulled inside the leg and is held at the flank region. The head is held firmly and the hind and fore legs are tied separately to avoid any pressure on the thorax and injury to the leg.

Reuff's Method

A loop is made around the animals neck or horn using a bow-line knot. The free end of the rope is thrown over the back to the opposite side. The end is picked up and brought around the body and under the standing part of the rope near the bowline to form a half hitch just behind the shoulder. Another half hitch is made by crossing the end of the rope over the animals back infront of the udder or prepuce. The rope is pulled to force the animals to lie down. The hind and forelimbs are then tied separately.

Casting a buffalo: Two ropes about 5 meter long are taken. With one end of a rope a clove hitch is applied on both forelimbs just above the fetlock after bringing the fore limbs together. A similar half hitch is applied to the hind limbs around the hind cannon just above the fetlock. The ends of the ropes are pulled to cast the animal. The animal is supported with hands on the side to which the animal is expected to fall to prevent injury. The tail is slipped through the hind limbs and is held by an assistant. The limbs are then tied together. Sufficient bedding is provided where casting restraint is done.

Other Methods

i) Flanking

ii) Tilt Tables

Precautions

a) The ground where the animal is to be casted should be soft and free from any sharp edged objects.

b) Normally, animal should be casted on right side except during pregnancy.

Assignments

a) Practice and write the procedure for application of all knots in general and milkman's knot, halter, straight jacket and casting ropes in particular. Also mention the length and thickness of ropes required.

b) Draw the diagrams of various equipments required for the above said exercise.

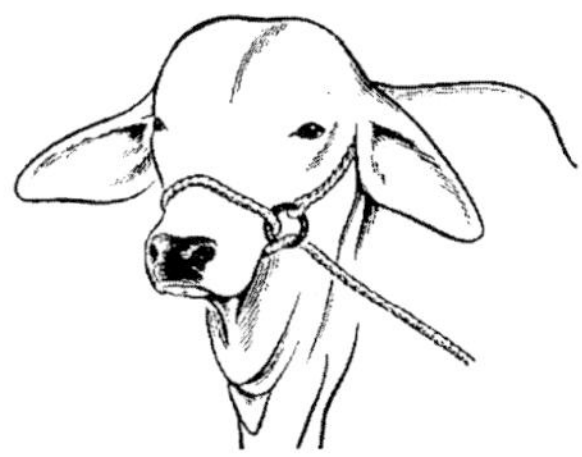

Halter

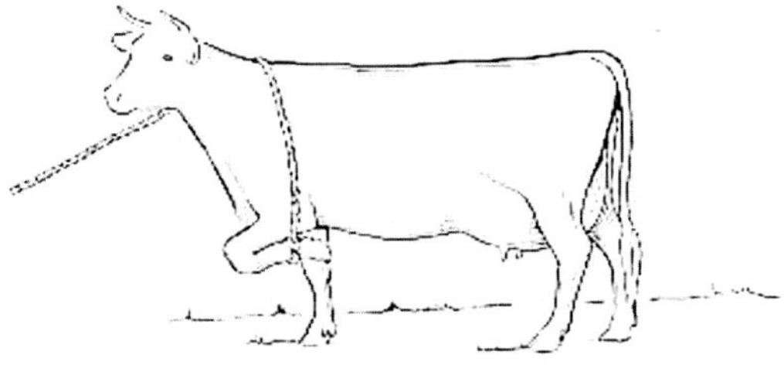

Lifting forelimb of animal

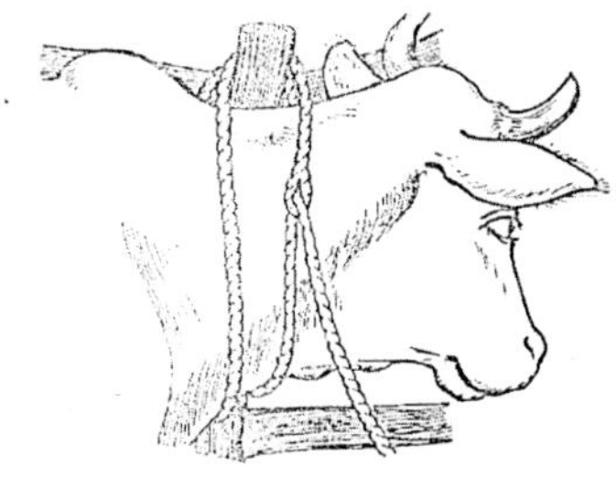

Dehorning restrain

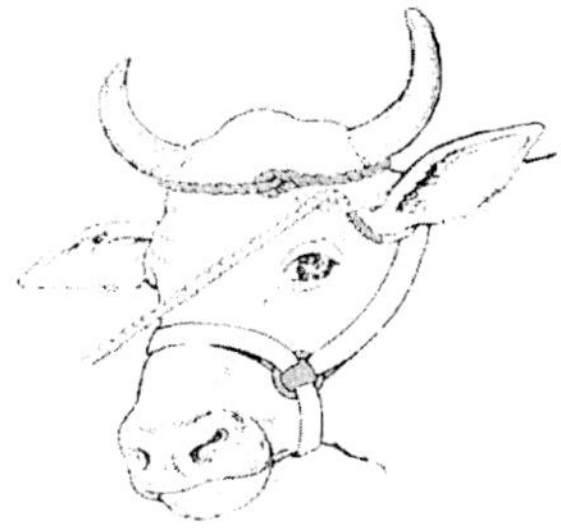

Ear twich

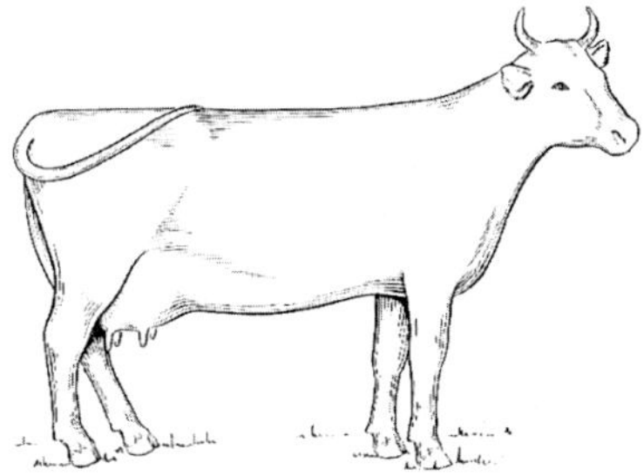

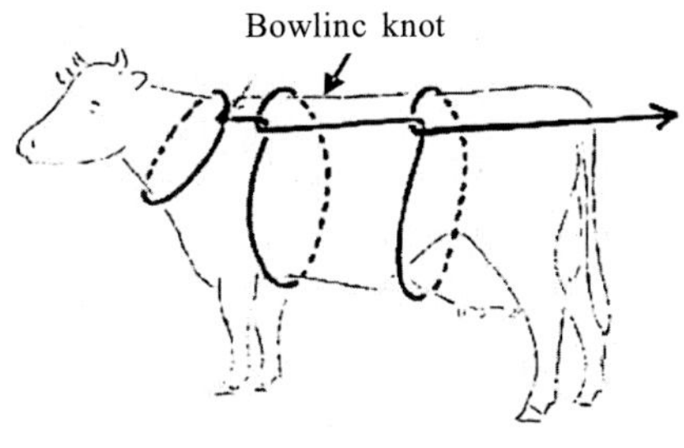

Reuff's method of casting

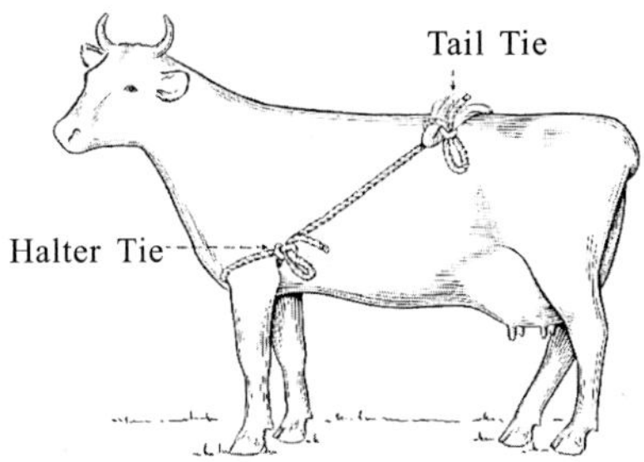

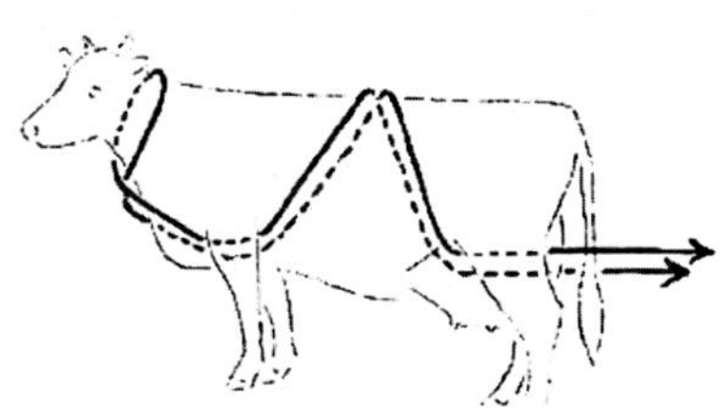

Alternate (Criss-crose) method of casting

Graphics Compiled and edited from Web Resource

Questions

a) Why do we use two ropes for handling of bulls?

b) Why bull nose ring is not used in case of cows?

c) How will you handle a bull when he has no nose ring?

d) Why milkman's knot is not generally applied in buffaloes?

e) In what case calf muzzle is applied?

f) What is tail twist?

Signature of Teacher

❑❑❑

22

Approaching, Handling and Restraining of Sheep and Goat

Date:

Objective

To approach, handle and restrain sheep and goat for different managemental practices to be carried on these species.

Material Required

Animals, ropes of different sizes, shepherd's crook, halter, chains, tethering pins, charts, figures and diagrams etc.

Procedure

Both sheep and goat are smaller ruminants. They can be easily handled. Whenever they are to be handled, first corner them and hold the required animal quickly and restrain its forward as well as rear movement by placing your hands on brisket or head on front side and flank or rump or buttocks on rear side.

Handling

1. Straddle Restraint:Holding the animal between the handler's legs while standing over the animal.

   Face parallel to the animal to examine mouth or for drenching, bolusing and balling.

   Face backward to examine the different organs and record rectal temperature etc.

2. Lifting of fore leg.

3. Lifting of rear leg

4. Casting by flanking method
5. Casting by criss-cross method
6. Set up position
7. Halter restraint

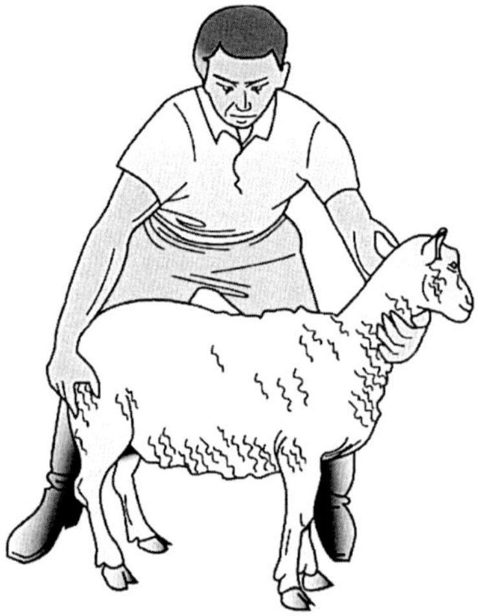

Holding a sheep

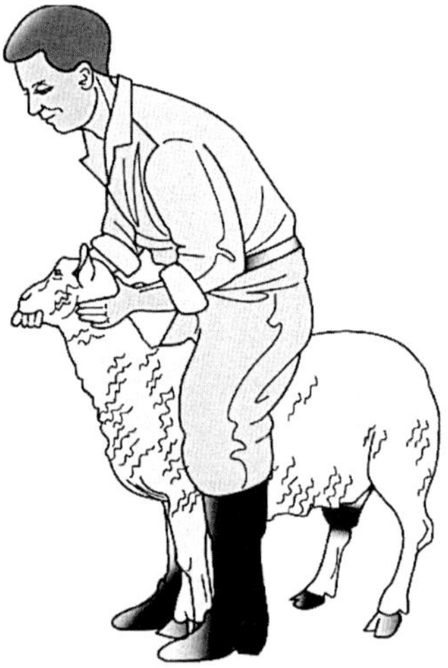

Straddle Restraint

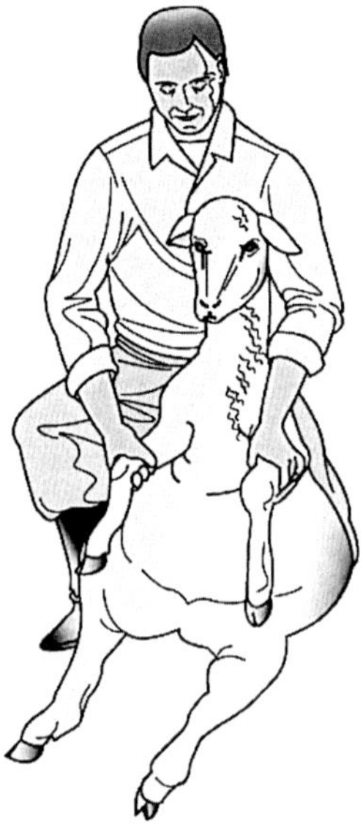

Hoof trimming

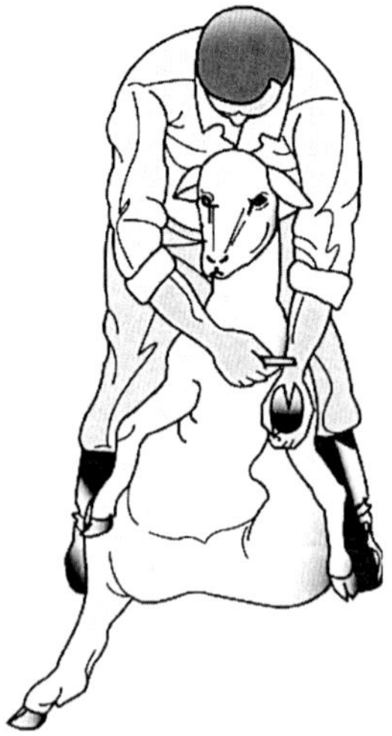

Hoof examination

Graphic Source : Web Resource

Precautions

i) Ensure that at the time of set up position, angle of the animal with ground is of 60^0.

ii) While dealing with goats, one should be very cautious.

iii) Normally, ruminants should be casted on the right side and there should not be any sharp article on the ground.

iv) Never throw the animal on ground, place it gently to avoid injury.

v) Never pull the sheep by holding its wool.

Assignments

i) Draw diagrams of different methods of restraining sheep and goat.

ii) Learn to make halter for sheep and goat.

Questions

i) Why goat can't be made to sit in set up position like sheep?

Signature of Teacher

❑❑❑

23

Dipping and Spraying of Sheep

Date:

Objective

1. For control of ectoparasites.
2. To cure or prevent sheep scab.
3. To ward off attack by sheep blow flies.
4. To remove waste material and dung from the fleece prior to shearing.

Time of dipping

Once a year either before post winter shearing or before post autumn shearing.

When there is high incidence of ectoparasites sheep can be dipped one month after shearing when the fleece has grown long enough to retain dip solution.

Dipping methods

1. Hand bath method
2. Swim bath method

Hand bath method

1. Used for small flock
2. The tank is constructed of wood or galvanised iron about 1.2m x 1.0m x 0.5m
3. Sheep are lifted one by one into the bath and kept for 2 minutes. The head should be immersed atleast once.

4. It is then lifted on to a draining board, where the surplus dip is squeezed from its fleece to go back into the bath.
5. Two men dip the sheep and one catches them.

Swim bath method

1. Used for large flock of sheep
2. The measurement of dipping tank depends on the number of sheep kept, but in general they are 1.5m deep, 2.5-3m long at the top, 1.5-2m long at the bottom and 1m wide.
3. They are made of concrete at the ground level or slightly raised. A collecting pen should be situated at one end of the draining pen at the other end of the bath. The draining pen should have a gradient towards the dip tank.
4. The sheep lowered into the deep end of the dip swim through and walks up the ramp into the draining pen. While swimming through the dip they may be guided and helped along by a man with a pole having a fork-shaped end.

Precautions to be taken before and after dipping

1. Always rest and water the sheep before dipping to avoid drinking ofdip solution.
2. Remove soiled and dung stained wool on the crutch by hand shear before dipping.
3. The dipping bath should be thoroughly cleaned few days before dipping.
4. The dipping material in the tank should be sufficient to submerge the animal.
5. The direction for use of medicine should be strictly followed.
6. The liquid should be maintained nearly at body temperature.
7. The bath should be thoroughly stirred from top to bottom.
8. Dipping should not be carried out in hot or cold or rainy weather. If necessary in rainy weather, water proofing dip may be used.
9. Dip solution should be prepared a day earlier.

10. Dipping should be commenced in bright days in the morning and completed at least 2-3 hours before evening to ensure proper drying.
11. Dip the lamb first, and then adult sheep and the lamb last.
12. Avoid dipping ram in breeding season to prevent injury to the penis or scalding of the thigh.
13. Ewes in advanced stage of pregnancy should not be dipped. If necessary they should be handled gently in small lot.
14. Do not dip sick animal, sheep with open wound, very young lamb and stock being sent for slaughter.
15. Do not use carbolic acid and tar preparation for sheep in full fleece to avoid staining and brittleness of wool fibres.
16. Do not dip sheep immediately or within 10 days of shearing rather about a month post shearing.
17. Allow sheep to stand for 15 min in the dripping tank before turning them out on pasture.
18. On completion of dipping, materials should be disposed off properly.

Spraying

The animals are tightly packed together in a room and insecticidal solution is sprayed along the back and sides in the form of fine mist.

Questions

1. Draw the structure of dipping tank.
2. Name the commonly used chemicals used for dipping.

Signature of Teacher

❑❑❑

24

Shearing of Sheep

Date:

Shearing is the removal of wool from the body of the sheep

Objective

1. To obtain wool easily and quickly without any injury to any part of the sheep.
2. To minimise discomfort to the shearer and sheep as well.

Materials required

1. Hand shears (For flock size less than 10 sheep)
2. Hand shears/clippers (For flock of 100 sheep)
3. Power shears/Clippers (For flock of more than 100 sheep)
4. Shearing board.

Time of shearing

a) Twice a year in plains
   i) At the end of winter season (March–April)
   ii) At the end of rainy season (Sept-Oct)
b) Thrice a year in hilly areas
   i) February- march
   ii) May-June
   iii) September-October

Preparing sheep for shearing

1. Sheep should be washed in running water 10-15 days before shearing to clean the wool. Waiting for 10-15 days helps in

returning some grease to the fleece. Greased fibres are stronger and they cut more easily and uniformly.

2. Sheep should not be fed for 10 hours before shearing to protect the fleece from the stains of manure excreted during shearing.
3. Individual sheep first should be cleaned of soiled wool and thorns.
4. Clip away urine and dung stained wool and keep it separate.
5. Sheep to be clipped should be placed on a smooth broad platform to obtain clean wool.
6. Sheep waiting for their turn should be kept in clean pen.

Shearing procedure

Two most common procedures are

i) **Along the sheep :** Shorn in parallel strokes from head to hindquarter. First on side is done with the sheep lying on one side of the body, then it is turned over and the other side is completed.

ii) **Around the sheep :** Done in circular strokes around the body. Sheep is first made to sit on its buttock, back away from the shearer and the wool is removed by strokes going round the sheep from the fleece opening at the throat, first around the neck, then around the shoulders, back and so on.

Different shearer prefers different methods and many uses combination of the two. Whatever method of shearing is adopted, it is necessary first to open the fleece. To open the fleece, sheep has to be reopened in sitting position by :

1. Standing at the left side and
2. Running your left hand under sheep's neck.
3. Running your right hand over the sheep, and catch the right flank.
4. Pulling up and back, sheep is set up.
5. To keep the hind feet off the floor- hold the sheep tilted back a little, supported against your leg.
6. In horned sheep control the head by holding horns.

For shearing along the sheep, most shearers prefer shearing board. A large canvas makes a good floor for shearing. Some shearers tie up the legs.

Precautions

1. Never try to pull the wool for shearing purpose as it may cause cuts on the skin.
2. Hold the sheep firmly to prevent kicking and struggling of sheep to prevent injuries.
3. Keep the skin tight in front of the shears.
4. Always turn the sheep from left to right to shear off wool from right to left.
5. Extra care should be taken to prevent cuts on the sheath, withers, teats, flank, ears etc.
6. Prevent mixing of dung, sand and other foreign matters with fleece.
7. Shearing should be carried out at the time when the climate not very hot or cold.

Shearing methods

1. Hand shearing-Average 25-30 sheep/day can be sheared by hand shearing.
2. Machine shearing- More than 150 sheep/day can be sheared by using machine shearer.
3. Chemical shearing-Animals are fed with 24 mg cyclophosphamide per kg body weight for 12 days. Wool is removed after 3 days starting from 12 days after drug administration.

Questions

1. What are the precautions to be undertaken to combat post shearing stress?
2. What are the features of chemical shearing?

Signature of Teacher

❑❑❑

25

Routine sheep and goat operations

Date:

Objective

To acquaint with the routine sheep and goat farm operations.

Procedure

Visiting the farm and observation of following operations:

Approximate time	Farm operations
7.00 AM	1.Counting the animals, check the sick animals for treatment if any. 2.Send the animals for grazing. 3.During breeding season the rams should be allowed along with the ewes for grazing. 4.Nursing mothers should be retained inside the pen with lambs.
8.00 AM	1.Feeding half of the daily concentrate ration to nursing ewes, fattening or market lambs. 2.Arrangement should be made for watering sheep on grazing lands.
8.30AM	1.Feed chopped green or dry fodder to penned sheep. 2.Cleaning of all the sheds and disposal/ conservation of manure.
9AM to 3PM	Special jobs namely shearing, vaccination, dehorning, identification of lambs, daily recording of data, buying and selling of animals. Initial grading and baling of wool, marketing wool, training of sheep for show.

	Note: The farm manager should plan various jobs in advance and as per the season and the market demand. Extra labour should be employed during dipping and shearing days.
4PM	1.Returning the sheep from grazing, counting and penning. 2.Check the animals for the grazing efficiency on to the flank region and alertness. 3.Many decisions have to be taken for the animals which are not showing the signs of active grazing. 4.Feeding the remaining half of the concentrate ration to nursing ewes and market lambs. 5.Feeding dry fodder and chopped green fodder to all animals. **Note:** In goat farms the milch goats should be milked once in the morning and once in the evening at convenient times.

Assignments

Visit to farm and note routine farm operations at different time of day.

Signature of Teacher

❐❐❐

26

Spotting of Sick Animals

Date:

Objective

1. To identify the diseased animals from healthy one.
2. To know the animal behaviour indicating illness.

Sl. no.	Parameter	Healthy animal		Sick animal
		Sheep	Goat	
1.	Look of animal	Alert		Dull
2.	Head	Raised		Bent downwards
3.	Eyes	Wide open, bright		Dull with white deposition at the corners
4.	Conjunctival mucous membrane	Normal		Pale or congested
5.	Nose	No discharge		Slimy discharge
6.	Movement	Active		Sluggish, lameness
7.	Response	Quick		Slow
8.	Faeces	Normal		Hard / loose, mucus/blood-stained, discolouration, dysentry
9.	Pulse (/min)	70-90	70-90	Increased
10.	Body temperature (°F)	102.4	103.8	Increased
11.	Respiration (/min)	12-30	12-30	Increased, difficult
12.	Grazing	Normal		Abnormal
13.	Rumination	Regular		Irregular
14.	Feed and water intake	Normal		Reduced
15.	Udder	Normal		May be swollen
16.	Skin	Healthy		Infected, external parasites

Procedure

Visiting the farm and observe the following signs and record necessary parameters of animal.

Assignments

Visit the farm and observe the following signs and record necessary parameters.

Signature of Teacher

❑❑❑

27

Visit to Nearby Wildlife Sanctuary/Zoo/Wild Animal Centre

Date:

Objective

1. To get familiarize with the different types of wild animals available at the centre.
2. To observe the care and management practices of different zoo animals.
3. To get familiarize with restraint examination of the different types of wild animals.
4. To observe the housing system of different zoo animals.

Material required

Wild animals of different species, Models, charts, diagrams of different species, different physical facilities and records/information on different species.

Procedure

After taking a round of the livestock farms tabulate the information as per guidelines given in the following sections:

1. Care and management practices of different zoo animals.
2. Restraint examination of the different types of wild animals.
3. Housing system of different zoo animals.

Precautions

1. Dip your feet in footbath, if provided.

2. Don't try to tease or provoke the animals.
3. Don't make noise while examining animal or animal premises.

Assignments

1. Describe physical descriptions/anatomy of your species.
2. Define any terminology deemed appropriate for your species.
3. Describe any specific laws/regulations of Central Zoo Authority (CZA) standards that are specific for your species.

Signature of Teacher

❑❑❑

28

Studying the Housing of Captive Animals

Date:

Objective

To assemble information on basic housing requirements, best practices, and animal care recommendations to maximize capacity for excellence in animal care and welfare.

Procedure

Tabulate the following information based on your observation:

A) Taxonomic Classification

Taxonomic classification for ....

Classification	Taxonomy	Additional information
Kingdom		
Phylum		
Class		
Order		
Suborder		
Family		

Genus, Species, and Status

Genus	Species	Common Name	India Status	IUCN Status

B) Ambient Environment

i) **Temperature and Humidity**

The animals must be protected or provided accommodation from weather, and any adverse conditions. Animals not normally exposed to cold weather/water temperatures should be provided heated enclosures/pool water. Likewise, protection from excessive cold weather/water temperatures should be provided to those animals normally living in warmer climates/water temperatures.

ii) **Light**

Careful consideration should be given to the spectral, intensity, and duration of light needs for all animals in the care of zoos and aquariums.

iii) **Water and Air Quality**

Zoos must have a regular program of monitoring water quality for aquatic animals, and a written record must document long-term water quality results and chemical additions. Monitoring selected water quality parameters provides confirmation of the correct operation of filtration and disinfection of the water supply available for the collection. Additionally, high quality water enhances animal health programs instituted for aquatic collections.

iv) **Sound and Vibration**

Consideration should be given to controlling sounds and vibrations that can be heard by animals in the care of zoos and aquariums.

C) Habitat Design and Containment

i) **Space and Complexity**

Careful consideration should be given to exhibit design so that all areas meet the physical, social, behavioral, and psychological needs of the species. Animals must be well cared for and presented in a manner reflecting modern zoological practices in exhibit design. All animals must be housed in safe enclosures that meet their physical and psychological needs, as well as their social needs.

ii) **Natural Appearance**

- The housing arrangements need to merge with the natural surroundings and this avoids the distraction when visitors see the enclosure. Hence, the objectives of visiting of zoos may be achieved.

- For many wild animal species, housing arrangements should include naturally simulating infrastructures and for example, trees may be placed`1/grown inside the arboreal species like nilgiri langur.
- The visible structural elements of the barriers that are in direct line of the vision of visitors andexhibit species should be painted suitably, so as to render those structuralelements to appear like those of local soil.

iii. Inside - over hangs as housing facility

- Overhangs are required particularly in case of animals that are capable of jumping to a great height. This helps to give protection to both visitors and wild animal species.
- Following wild animal species need the inside-overhangs in general:

Cheetah	Sambar deer	• Impala
Zebra	Mouse deer	• Chinkara
Wild ass	Musk deer	• Nilgiri tahr
Spotted deer	Brow antlered deer	
Hog deer	Four horned antelope	

iv) **Floor of mammalian enclosure**

- In case of elephants, the floor arrangements should not be made only by concrete.
- Natural substrate has to be provided to avoid the foot rot. Similarly, for cervids and antelopes, natural floor is a must.
- Avoid the presence of any pointed materials during the construction of the housing arrangements.
- Drainage facilities need to be provided while designing the floor arrangements inside the mammalian or other enclosures.
- Flooring arrangement needs to be made in order to facilitate an easy cleaning of the premises. Crevices need to be taken care of during theroutine management.

v) **Floor of Aviaries**

- Care has to be taken to protect the aviary species from the predators that use the floor or sides, often. Hence, the aviary enclosure or housing arrangement needs to be intelletually established, considering many features required by avi fauna of multiple species, in general.

- Rodent control is an important measure for the wild birds that are kept in the confined state.
- Floors of aviaries should have cement concrete floors in order to prevent the entry of rodents and have to be topped by the layer of about 15 cms earth.

vi) **Floor of reptilian houses**

- The reptilian houses should have land as well as the water-designs that should allow the sufficient space for both bathing and basking.
- The substrate for the reptile cages should be of pea-sized gravel or sand materialdepending upon the species of the reptiles.

vii) **Doors**

The doors of any wild animal species should be constructed considering the following factors in mind:

- Safety (Secured locking systems must be provided in order to prevent the theft or vandalism and to prevent the unauthorized opening of the cages in which the wild animals have been kept in confined status)
- Durability
- Easy handling nature
- Gilletin type of vertical doors are to be avoided and horizontally, sliding doors may be used with proper lock-positions.

Anatomy and Housing Arrangements

- The entry door of the enclosure has to be constructed in a careful manner in order to avoid the injuries to the wild animal.
- The opening has to be an adequate one, so that the concerned wild animal species can make entry freely into the enclosure.
- The entry door of the wild animal species like Giraffe has to be built so high enough to accommodate the long neck of this animal.

- Elephant should enter into the enclosure freely without any struggles and the housing arrangement has to be done in such a manner that entry related difficulties have to be avoided in general.

Nature of the Species and Housing

The nature of the concerned wild animal species has to be given more significance whenever a proper housing arrangement is made.

- Chimpanzees generally are reluctant to approach the water resources except for the drinking purposes. Hence, wet moats are generally preferred ones whenever housing arrangements are made for them.
- Giraffe do not swim and hence will not have inclination to cross the water moat. Further, the Giraffe are generally reluctant to step over the barriers and also have been very rarely observed to step over the shallow ditch. Similarly, Giraffe can extend the neck to a great extent during the attempting of trying to receive food material if any given by visitor. Hence, during the construction of housing facilities for species like this, all considerations have to be given to such nature of this species.
- Wet moats with resting platforms appear to be the must in case of housing arrangements for felids like tigers.

Feeding Place and Housing

- The place for feeding should be constructed in such a manner that the cleaning of the premises becomes an easy one and the crevices in the feeding trough needs to be attended properly during the maintenance of the feeding trough or place. This helps to avoid the deposition of feed particles in the structures and thereby thechances for contamination of food particles get minimized.
- Multiple feeding places are the better ones especially for the animals that are exhibited inherds like Spotted deer, Manipuri deer, black bucks etc.

Watering and Foot Bath Arrangements

- The watering facility should be thought of whenever a housing facility is constructed for the concerned wild animal species.

- The capacity of wild animal species with regard to the watering habits needs to be paid more emphasis.
- For example, an elephant may require about two hundred and twenty litres of water in a day.
- Hence, the watering trough should be of adequate size and should have an easy access for the wild animal species to have waterwhenever it desires.
- These need to be constructed outsidethe enclosure and by placing appropriate agents, it becomes possible to preventor minimize the entry of microbes through the visiting personnel.
- Place of foot bath should beinspected frequently to avoid the slippery nature of the floor.

Name of the Species	**Size of the cubicle in meters**		
	Length	**Breadth**	**Height**
Tiger and lions	2.75	1.80	3.00
Panther	2.00	1.50	2.00
Clouded leopard & snow leopard	2.00	1.50	2.00
Small cats	1.80	1.50	1.50
Elephant	8.00	6.00	5.50
One-horned Indian Rhinoceros	5.00	3.00	2.50
Brow antlered deer	3.00	2.00	2.50
Hangul	3.00	2.00	2.50
Swamp deer	3.00	2.00	2.50
Musk deer	2.50	1.50	2.00
Mouse deer	1.50	1.00	1.50
Nilgiri tahr	2.50	1.50	2.00
Chinkara	2.50	1.50	2.00
Four horned antelope	2.50	1.50	2.00
Wild Buffalo	3.00	1.50	2.00
Gaur	3.00	2.00	2.50

Name of the Species	Size of the cubicle in meters		
	Length	Breadth	Height
Yak	4.00	2.00	2.50
Bharal, goral, Wild sheep and markhor	2.50	1.50	2.00
Wild Ass	4.00	2.00	2.00
All type of Indian bears	2.50	1.80	2.00
Jackal, wolf and Wild dog	2.00	1.50	1.50
Palm civet	2.00	1.00	1.00
Large Indian civet & binturong	2.00	1.50	1.00
Otters all types	2.50	1.50	1.00
Hogbadger	2.50	1.50	1.00
Martens	2.00	1.50	1.00
Red Panda	3.00	1.50	1.00
Slow loris and slender loris	1.00	1.00	1.50
Macaques and langurs	2.00	1.00	1.50

ii) **Safety and Containment**

Animals housed in free-ranging environments should be carefully selected, monitored and treated humanely so that the safety of these animals and persons viewing them is ensured. Animal exhibits and holding areas must be secured to prevent unintentional animal egress. All animal exhibit and holding area air and water inflows and outflows must also be securely protected to prevent animal injury or egress.

Common barriers

Common six types of barriers thatare generally used in case of captive wild animal places are given below:

- Glass panels
- Plastic panels
- Wire-mesh fencing or chain link fences
- Wet and dry moats of adequate dimension
- High tensile vertical wires

- Electrically charged wires
- Concrete barriers in selected sides

Stand-off barriers

- The enclosure barriers are themust and more cautions need to be exercised in order to design these types of barriers especially for the hazardous type of wild animal species like tiger,panther, lion, jaguar etc.

Spread out of the railing beyond barriers

- If there is a direct contact between the wild animal species and the visitor, then there are chances for the visitors to get injured by the highly capable animals like lions, tiger etc.
- Hence, there is an immediate requirement to construct the stand-off barrier like the construction of Spaced-Out railing beyond the barriers which help top revent any accidental contact with the concerned wild animal species.

Security of Fences

- More care has to be paid in the construction of the fences that has security related features.
- If not, the visitors as well as the wild animal species may get injured. Particular attention is to be given to protect the children also during the visit to the captive wild animal places.
- The barriers should not injure the children or anybody.
- Describe monitoring mechanisms and protocols of your species.
- Describe containment recommendations for animals used in conservation and education programs, especially those involving close contact with visitors (e.g., walk-through aviaries and yards where the zoo visitor is routinely in the animal enclosure).
- Exhibits in which the visiting public is not intended to have contact with animals must have a barrier of sufficient strength and/or design to deter such contact.

Assignments

- ❒ Recommend specific climate control equipment & facilities needed for your species.
- ❒ Recommend air/water testing protocols and equipment if needed.
- ❒ Identify potential sources of sound/vibration problems that may be caused within and outside environments (e.g., construction, pumps, filtration, generators, cleaning machines).
- ❒ Define appropriate means of measuring, addressing, and controlling sound stimuli, if any.

Questions

- ❒ Describe appropriate exhibit space and complexity recommendations needed to meet the needs of your species, promote species-appropriate behaviors and provide for appropriate socialization.
- ❒ Define inter-individual distances needed for your species (social hierarchies, etc.).
- ❒ Describe guardrail/barrier recommendations for your species if appropriate.

Signature of Teacher

❒❒❒